WHAT NURSES KNOW . . .

MULTIPLE
SCLEROSIS

WHAT NURSES KNOW ...

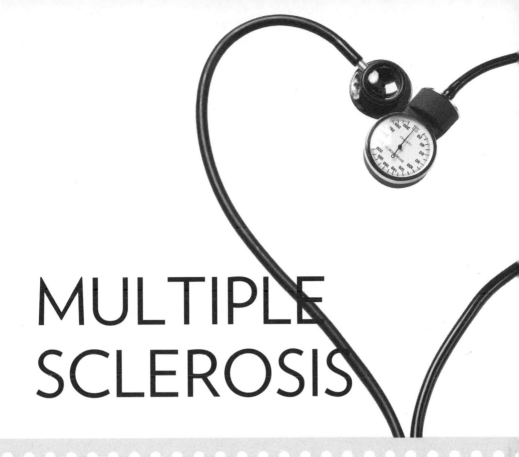

MULTIPLE SCLEROSIS

Carol Saunders
BA, BSN, MSCN

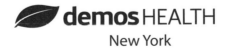

demos HEALTH

New York

Visit our web site at www.demoshealth.com

Acquisitions Editor: Noreen Henson
Cover Design: Steve Pisano
Compositor: NewGen
Printer: Hamilton Printing

Library of Congress Cataloging-in-Publication Data

Saunders, Carol.
   What nurses know—multiple sclerosis / Carol Saunders.
      p. cm.–(What nurses know)
   Includes index.
   ISBN 978-1-932603-89-7 (pbk.)
   1. Multiple sclerosis–Popular works. I. Title. II. Title: Multiple sclerosis.
   RC377.S2525 2911
   616.8'34–dc22   2010052239

Special discounts on bulk quantities of Demos Health books are available to corporations, professional associations, pharmaceutical companies, health care organizations, and other qualifying groups. For details, please contact:

Special Sales Department
Demos Medical Publishing
11 W. 42nd Street
New York, NY 10036
Phone: 800-532-8663 or 212-683-0072
Fax: 212-941-7842
E-mail: rsantana@demosmedpub.com

Made in the United States of America
11 12 13 14   5 4 3 2 1

About the Author

Carol Saunders, BA, BSN, MSCN, was the Director of Patient Care at the Neurology Center of Fairfax, Virginia. She has been a member of the Consortium of MS Centers since 1990, and a member of the International Organization of MS Nurses since its founding in 1997. Carol formerly served on the Professional Advisory Committee and Chapter Services Committee of the National Capital Area Chapter of the National Multiple Sclerosis Society (NMSS) and was a cofounder of the Greater Washington, DC, area Consortium of MS Nurses. She has been a member of the NMSS since 1993 and in 1998 was honored as the NMSS Volunteer of the Year. She has been a nurse for 25 years specializing in MS issues.

WHAT NURSES KNOW...

Nurses hold a critical role in modern health care that goes beyond their day-to-day duties. They share more information with patients than any other provider group, and are alongside patients twenty-four hours a day, seven days a week, offering understanding of complex health issues, holistic approaches to ailments, and advice for the patient that extends to the family. Nurses themselves are a powerful tool in the healing process.

What Nurses Know gives down-to-earth information, addresses consumers as equal partners in their care, and explains clearly what readers need to know and wants to know to understand their condition and move forward with their lives.

Contents

Foreword

What Nurses Know...Multiple Sclerosis is a very unusual book, one that provides all those affected by multiple sclerosis (MS) with a unique perspective, information from a vital member of the MS team, the MS nurse. Written by a woman who has had vast experience as an MS nursing professional, it has a unique format, a conversational tone that depicts quite accurately the persona of the author who is a very unusual leader and nursing role model. Each chapter is clearly written about topics of great importance to patients and their families: the definition of MS, symptomatic management, disease modifying therapies, treating exacerbations, and complementary therapies. In addition, vignettes are interspersed throughout the book with stories of real patients facing real challenges related to their disease. Call out boxes are placed in key areas entitled "What Nurses Know" containing highlights from the text. This is a very clever way of pointing out important things to remember from each chapter.

Each chapter is written on a personal level, just as if Carol were talking to her patients and their families. Carol's writing style resembles how she has interacted with patients and families throughout the years. It is as if she were counseling and educating them as she has been known to do. The information she provides is accurate and up-to-date and written in a very user-friendly manner. It is also the type of book that one can read through, bookmark, and revisit again to relearn and remind oneself about managing their multiple sclerosis.

This book is also a valuable teaching/learning tool for nursing professionals who can add to their body of knowledge about multiple sclerosis by reading it to enhance personal knowledge. It also can be used to educate patients and their families about particular topics. The case vignettes have an insight and poignancy that embody the author's style and personality: warm and caring. It is very unusual for a book such as this to allow the reader to sense this especially when dealing with medical diagnoses and treatments.

What Nurses Know...Multiple Sclerosis will be a valuable addition to our compendium of multiple sclerosis references. It will add to the body of resources of patients, families, and all those affected by multiple sclerosis. It also gives a voice to the role of MS nursing and to the importance of professional partnerships throughout the spectrum of this complex disease.

—June Halper, MSN, APN-C, FAAN, MSCN

Preface

You have seen a doctor who has told you that you have, probably have, may have, or do have multiple sclerosis (MS). You probably feel overwhelmed. You may have heard MS mentioned, but you have never had reason to know anything about it, or you may have seen things you didn't want to know. What you do know is that this is something that you probably would not choose to have. Now you will be forced to know about it. What is this going to mean in your life?

Not too many years ago when I, a nurse who works with MS patients, would go in to see someone who had been told that he or she had MS and I asked what that person knew about MS, he or she would often answer that Jerry Lewis had a weekend drive for money for MS every September on Labor Day weekend. I would know right away that this person knew nothing about MS. Jerry Lewis's drive benefits muscular dystrophy, a disease very unlike MS. We needed to start at the beginning. Today when I ask patients what they know about MS, they have been on the Internet and I am more likely to get two things: an answer saying that people with MS end up in wheelchairs and a look that says "Please don't say that I have that."

In this book I am going to discuss what MS is, and what it is not, and how people can live very full and meaningful lives with a diagnosis of MS. MS is a chronic condition, and it will be with you for your lifetime. It will present challenges that you may not have encountered if MS had not entered your life, but in meeting those challenges you will learn positive actions to take so you can manage this unexpected intrusion into your life and to improve that life.

Information and knowledge about MS are exploding. There are now a variety of medications that can make a real difference with MS, and many more are on the horizon. Health care professionals are able to provide comprehensive management for people with MS that goes beyond disease and symptom management. We want you to have all the information and support possible to empower you to live your life to its fullest.

—Carol Saunders, BA, BSN, MSCN

WHAT NURSES KNOW...

MULTIPLE
SCLEROSIS

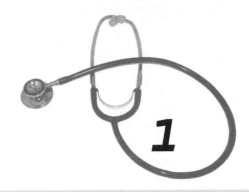

Multiple Sclerosis: What Is It?

I knew there was a disease called multiple sclerosis because I remember ads on TV asking for people to walk for people who had multiple sclerosis, but I had no reason to know anything about it. Then I just about lost my vision and my eye doctor sent me to a neurologist and I was told that I had multiple sclerosis. I guess I really need to know about it now.   MARLA

Back thirty-five years ago when I was just a little girl visiting my grandmother we would visit her friend who was in a wheelchair. My grandmother said that her friend had multiple sclerosis. Now I have multiple sclerosis and am scared. I need to know what it is and what my life will be like now.   PEGGY

Multiple sclerosis (MS) is a chronic disease. It is a condition that results from abnormal activity of the body's immune system and affects the central nervous system (CNS). It is most commonly diagnosed in young adults in their 20s and 30s—at least fifty percent of people with MS are diagnosed between age 20 and 40 years of age–although it is now being noted in children and often is seen in older adults. Older adults in looking back at their health history can point to earlier symptoms that may have been symptoms of MS. According to most publications on MS, there are at least 400,000 individuals with the disease in the United States, with at least an estimated 10,000 cases diagnosed per year, and 2.5 million individuals with MS worldwide. It is the most common neurological disorder among young adults and occurs approximately three times more frequently in women than in men. It is diagnosed more often in Caucasians than in Hispanics and African Americans, although in the "melting pot" of the United States it is noted in all populations. MS is said to be more common in temperate areas distant from the equator. It is most common in Canada and the northern United States, Great Britain, Scandinavia, Australia, and the southern parts of South America (Halper J. & Holland N. 1997 and van den Noort S. & Holland N. 1999).

MS is a demyelinating disease that affects the CNS, which comprises the brain and spinal cord. Nerves are made up of *neurons*, which have *dendrites*, branched filaments that are attached to neurons. The dendrites contain the cell's body and axons that are covered with *myelin*, a fatty substance that

What Nurses Know...

Studies show that the farther away you are from the equator the more likely you will be to develop MS; therefore, areas like Canada, the northern United States, and northern Europe have the highest population of people living with MS. However, as global populations continue to move and mix, other ethnic groups are "catching up."

functions as an insulating material, like the covering on an electrical wire. Neurons transmit impulses to and from the brain, and myelin allows these impulses to be transmitted rapidly and smoothly. In MS, areas of myelin are destroyed and become scarred, and because there are many scarred or sclerotic areas or lesions the condition is named *multiple sclerosis*, which means "many scars." Inflammation occurs where the myelin is attacked, and because of this inflammation impulses are not transmitted in the brain or spinal cord at the rate they were before, and MS symptoms result. When the inflammation subsides, impulses once again are transmitted at the same rate as before (or almost as fast as before) and symptoms resolve, or at least abate. MS can be difficult to diagnose early in the course of the disease, because the symptoms often come and go as just described. Early in the disease, some regeneration of the neuron's myelin sheath can occur, and once again impulses are transmitted at the same rate, or nearly the same rate, and symptoms disappear. However, the axon that was covered by the myelin can degenerate, and when that happens impulses can no longer be transmitted and symptoms do not improve. Progressive axonal loss may explain the brain atrophy, or tissue loss, that occurs later in the disease. This tissue loss can be noted with the help of magnetic resonance imaging (MRI).

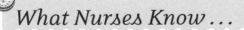

What Nurses Know...

It is helpful to know other people who have MS and compare notes. You may have some of the same symptoms. But you can't look at someone else and figure that your disease course will be just like that person's, because no two people with MS are exactly alike.

MS is an autoimmune disease in which, for some unknown reason, the body's own immune system attacks normal myelin. Symptoms result from this inflammatory process and from the ensuing damage to the axons. These attacks are insidious and not predictable, which means that the course of the disease itself is not predictable, which is one of the most difficult aspects of having MS. Unpredictability can be hard for everyone, because we all like to feel that we are in control. No two people with MS are exactly alike, because these attacks on myelin can occur anywhere in the CNS. Different areas of the brain and spinal cord are responsible for different kinds of movements, and a person's symptoms depend on the exact location of the attack that is causing a lesion.

You probably think of your immune system as the system that is responsible for destroying foreign substances, such as bacteria or viruses. MS is considered an autoimmune disorder because the immune system is too active: It sends out specific types of white blood cells that attack myelin as though it were a foreign substance.

MS is not a hereditary disease; however, although no specific gene for MS has been identified, several researchers have concluded that people with MS inherit certain regions on individual chromosomes more often than people without MS. About ten to twenty percent of people with MS are able to locate people with MS in their extended families, a higher rate than one

What Nurses Know...

There are many other autoimmune diseases you may have heard of, ranging from rheumatoid arthritis, to Graves' disease, to lupus. Even type 1 diabetes is an autoimmune disorder.

would expect by chance. Therefore, even though people do not inherit MS, they may inherit the *possibility* of developing MS. In the general population there is about a 0.2 percent (1:2,000) chance of developing the disease. If a parent has MS the probability of his or her daughter developing the disease is four percent (4:100), and the probability of that parent's son will develop MS is two percent (2:100). In identical twins, if one twin has MS there is a thirty percent chance that the other twin will have it, too. If MS were an inherited disease, that chance would be one hundred percent. MS is a multifactorial disease, meaning there are more than one factor involved in its cause, and all of the factors must interact in a specific way to result in the disease. Many investigators believe that a virus may be responsible for making the immune system act in an abnormal fashion and cause MS to develop, although so far no specific viruses have been consistently isolated. Research on MS is progressing at a remarkable rate, with more potential therapies in the pipeline than at any other time in history.

Diagnosing MS is anything but easy. There is no specific test for it. Often, getting an MS diagnosis is a process of eliminating all other possibilities. People who have finally been diagnosed with definite MS will typically have been through several medical professionals and maybe even several different diagnoses. Your doctor will start with a very complete history of your health and then will order an MRI of your head and neck, some evoked potential studies (that measure the rate and form of nerve impulses) and perhaps a spinal tap or lumbar puncture, as well as many

What Nurses Know...

Nothing you did caused you to have MS. Do not blame yourself!

What Nurses Know...

When MS is in its early stages, symptoms can be hard to interpret; also, they seem come and go. This makes it very difficult to diagnose. A lot of people are given a possible diagnosis as part of a "wait and see" approach, which can be very anxiety provoking.

laboratory tests, to rule out other causes of the symptoms you have. I discuss these tests in detail in Chapter 2.

Getting to a formal diagnosis of MS can be a long and complicated process. There may be anxiety-provoking misdiagnoses along the way. When you know that something is wrong, and that that "something" is serious, you experience a great fear of the unknown. This is normal. Many people confess to being terrified during the diagnosis stage, even more than when they are finally diagnosed.

I am 25 years old. I am a chemical engineer and I landed a super job that I love. I have wonderful friends and have been playing soccer on a team where I work. I have always been a jock. Lately I have not been an asset to the team. My left leg is weak, and last week I took a really bad fall. I was taken to the [emergency room] to rule out an injury to my head. After an MRI, the doc there told me that I needed to see a neurologist as it looked like I could have multiple sclerosis. I have seen multiple sclerosis on health forms that I have filled out, and I always check "no." I'll make an appointment with a neurologist, and I guess I had better learn something about multiple sclerosis.   WARREN

Classifications of Multiple Sclerosis

There are four different types of MS: (a) relapsing-remitting, (b) secondary progressive, (c) primary progressive, and (d) progressive-relapsing (see the Figure below). It is believed that eighty-five percent of MS cases begin as relapsing-remitting, in which acute attacks occur with either full recovery or some remaining symptoms and residual deficit. The periods between relapses show stability and no disease progression. Over time the course of the disease may change, and it may become progressive. In secondary progressive MS the relapsing-remitting form of the disease develops a more consistently progressive course, and although there may be occasional relapses and minor remissions permanent disability occurs. At least fifty percent of relapsing-remitting patients develop secondary progressive MS when not treated.

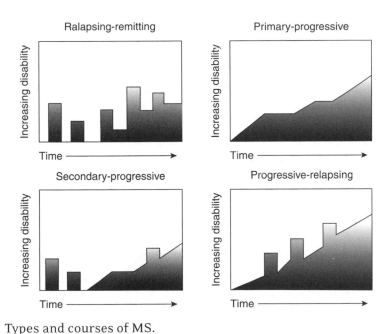

Types and courses of MS.

Fortunately, immunotherapy treatments are changing this picture. The third type of MS, primary progressive, occurs in perhaps ten percent of the MS population and is characterized by progression of disability from diagnosis on. It has no obvious remissions, although there may be occasional plateaus and temporary minor improvements. A small percentage of people, perhaps five percent, may have progressive-relapsing MS. In this type of MS there is significant recovery immediately following a relapse, but between relapses there is a gradual worsening of symptoms overall.

These four MS classifications were put into place before medications that could make a difference became available. These are discussed further in Chapter 3. The prognosis of MS can look very different thanks to new treatments; for example, many patients diagnosed with relapsing-remitting MS do not advance to secondary progressive MS. Patients who have been diagnosed with MS often want to know what classification they are in, but despite the fact that four separate classifications have been identified it is really impossible to categorize anyone into a definite class. What people want to hear is that they have what used to be termed *benign MS*, which allows a person to remain fully functional in all neurologic systems without relapses and without progression for at least fifteen years. However, as researchers learned more about MS they realized that there is probably no such thing as a "benign" form of the disease. Damage can occur in the CNS even when symptoms are not present. For a person diagnosed with MS, however, it is very important to know that most people with MS have a normal life span. For people who do have a progressive form of MS, the progression usually stops at some point; probably twenty percent of patients remain fairly stable. More aggressive disease management helps the other eighty percent have an satisfactory lifestyle and an acceptable quality of life.

Symptoms of MS vary widely, depending on the location of the affected nerve fibers. It is not surprising that a disease that damages the CNS can produce a very wide range of symptoms.

What Nurses Know ...

In recent years researchers have found that most MS is not as progressively disabling as once thought. This runs counter to common wisdom that MS as a disease marked by a steady decline in motor function. MS is not a progressive disease that inevitably leads to a wheelchair.

Indeed, there are few diseases with more potential symptoms than MS. The most common symptoms of MS are

- Fatigue
- Depression
- Cognitive issues
- Bladder dysfunction
- Numbness and/or tingling in the extremities
- Sexual dysfunction
- Bowel dysfunction
- Pain
- Dizziness and vertigo
- Muscle spasticity
- Tremor
- Vision problems

As you can see from this list, which includes only some of the symptoms of MS, the symptoms are varied and far reaching. As the disease progresses, more symptoms appear, and existing symptoms can get worse. I discuss these MS symptoms and how they are managed in Chapter 4.

Because MS affects the CNS, and the CNS governs almost every system in the body, this disease can cause a wide range of symptoms that in turn make it difficult to diagnose. If you suspect you might have MS, the first thing you need to do is to make certain that your symptoms don't have another cause that is not MS. Again, there is no one test that can verify that you definitely have MS, so your health care practitioner must first rule out everything else. If you are diagnosed with MS, your health care practitioner will treat your symptoms and introduce you to medications that can help alleviate the symptoms of the disease.

References

Halper J. & Holland N. (1997). Comprehensive Nursing Care in Multiple Sclerosis, New York, Demos Vermande, 1-3.

van den Noort S. & Holland N. (1999). Multiple Sclerosis in Clinical Practice, New York, Demos, 1-2.

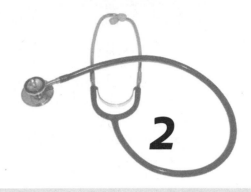

2

How Is Multiple Sclerosis Diagnosed?

I went to my doctor because I noticed numbness in my legs and a tingling feeling in my legs. He sent me to see a neurologist, saying that I might have multiple sclerosis. How will the neurologist know if that is what I have?   MITCH

Back in 1985, while I was playing football in college, my right leg became very weak and I had to stop playing. None of the doctors I saw could find a reason for my problem, and in a month or so I was back to normal. A year later my left arm did the same thing, and one of the doctors said I might have multiple sclerosis but there was nothing that could be done about it if I did and I did get better. I have had other symptoms since that time, and then last month I was unable to walk at all. This time, I was put into the hospital and had lots of tests, and I do have multiple sclerosis. I am grateful to have a name for my symptoms and a reason for them. We have come a long way in the last twenty-five years.   PHIL

If you have been diagnosed with multiple sclerosis (MS), you have in all probability gone to your doctor with symptoms that may be motor, sensory, or cognitive in nature. You may complain of increased fatigue; numbness or tingling in your legs and/or hands; and visual disturbances, such as double vision, blurred vision, or loss of vision. Perhaps your problem is related to balance or coordination, weakness or increased fatigue, or bowel and bladder dysfunction. In looking for a cause of your problem, your doctor may suspect that it is neurological or even that you have MS and refer you to a neurologist.

The first thing that a neurologist will do is take a detailed history, including your symptoms and complaints, your general health, and your family history. That will be followed by a thorough physical and neurological examination in which the neurologist looks for conditions that might explain the symptoms you are experiencing or to see if you have other symptoms of which you are unaware. Your eyes will be checked with an ophthalmoscope so the neurologist can observe your optic nerve for evidence of double vision or uncoordinated eye movements. Your coordination will be tested with a finger-to-nose test and heel-to-shin test. You will likely be asked to walk on your toes, and then on your heels, and then in tandem (walking in a straight line with toes touching your heels as you walk) and to stand with your eyes closed to check your balance. You'll be checked for sensory changes with a vibrating instrument. Your reflexes will be checked, and a number of tests will be performed that may help confirm the diagnosis of MS or to rule out other problems that might be causing your symptoms. There is still no one test that confirms a definite diagnosis of MS; it remains a clinical diagnosis made by a physician on the basis of symptoms and test results. The neurologist should share with you the results of your tests and explain the reasons why he or she feels you have a definite diagnosis of MS, a probable diagnosis of MS, or a possible diagnosis of MS.

You will need a health care team composed of individuals with whom you feel comfortable and confident. It is important that you have a good relationship with your primary medical doctor, who will remain a very important member of your health care team. The importance of wellness in your life cannot be stressed too much. It is so easy, once you have a diagnosis of a chronic condition such as MS, to blame everything else that happens to you on that diagnosis. Unfortunately, having MS does not exempt you from having other physical conditions as well. Your primary medical doctor is likely an internist, general practitioner, or family practitioner who deals with many complicated medical problems but does not specialize in MS. Neurologists are physicians who specialize in diseases of the central nervous system, and they usually manage MS along with their neurological team of nurse practitioners, physician's assistants, and nurses. Your primary medical doctor will continue to monitor your general health. Feel free to get a second opinion. Find a medical team that feels right to you. Do some research, and ask for recommendations; this is all within your rights as a patient. Your neurologist will want you to feel sure of your diagnosis and will see to it that you have your test results ready to present for a second opinion.

Magnetic Resonance Imaging

You will be sent to have a magnetic resonance imaging scan (MRI). For a definite diagnosis of MS, you will need to have plaques or lesions in at least two distinct areas in the myelin of your central nervous system. These plaques need to have formed at different points in time and must have no other reasonable explanation. MRIs have come a long way since they first became available in the 1990s. Pictures taken then looked like something taken with an old Brownie camera compared with the images of today. Today, the magnets in the machines are much stronger and capable of producing clear images that will be able to answer more questions. At the MRI center you will lie on a table that will move into a tube-like space in a large machine that holds the magnet. You must lie very still, and you will hear lots of noise as the magnet sends information to a computer that generates pictures that look like slices of your brain and spinal cord. The pictures are taken first without dye, to show total lesions, and then using a contrast dye called *gadolinium*, to highlight active lesions. There is no pain associated with the MRI procedure, but being in a closed and narrow space may cause claustrophobia. If claustrophobia is a problem for you, tell your doctor, and you can be given a prescription for Valium or Xanax to take before the procedure. If you do take a sedative, you must have a driver to bring you to the MRI center and drive you home, because these drugs can make you very sleepy. "Open MRIs" are available, but the pictures they produce are not as high quality as those in the closed MRI, and you likely will want the best pictures possible for your physician to view. Unfortunately, in the early stages of MS, if only a few minor symptoms are present an MRI may not always provide conclusive results. Alternatively, it may show changes that may or may not indicate MS, and you may need to repeat the procedure at a later date. Your physician will be looking for lesions caused by destruction of myelin and noting the locations of these lesions.

You may be surprised to know that, despite its accuracy, an MRI scan alone cannot be used to make a definite diagnosis of MS. Clinical symptoms are usually necessary and, because there are a number of other demyelinating conditions, these must be

What Nurses Know...

MRIs are painless and noninvasive procedures that provide lots of information. For identification of brain scarring or tumors there is nothing better. Unlike a computerized axial tomography scan (CT scan), it does not expose individuals to the hazards of ionizing radiation.

What Nurses Know...

MRI scans do not always pick up MS lesions. Some older lesions remyelinate sufficiently to be undetectable with an MRI scan.

ruled out. Your health care team may think your symptoms are being caused by MS but will also want evidence that there have been at least two identified demyelinating episodes separated by at least one month in at least two different locations in the central nervous system.

My doctor's office scheduled me for an MRI, and once I got there for it I just couldn't go through with it. I had never had reason to be claustrophobic before, but this was something else! My doctor prescribed some Xanax for me to take, and I tried again. This time, I just slept through the whole thing, and then a friend drove me home and I finished sleeping knowing that I had been able to have the MRI that was needed.   MIKE

Evoked Potentials

One test your physician may order is an *evoked potential study.* If the myelin sheath of neurons is damaged (demyelination), then nerve impulses are conducted more slowly than normal. Evoked potentials measure the rate and form of the impulse as it passes through specific nerves. Impulses on each side of the body can be compared to see if there is a slowing on one side. *Visual evoked potentials* check your visual system, *brain stem evoked potentials* look for lesions in the brain stem, and

What Nurses Know...

Evoked potential studies are painless and noninvasive and do not carry any significant risk. Somatosensory evoked potential tests involve very mild electric shocks, usually felt as a tingling.

somatosensory evoked potentials show changes in the extremities. Evoked potential studies are useful in confirming a diagnosis of MS.

Cerebrospinal Fluid

You may be asked to have a lumbar puncture, also called a *spinal tap* to confirm your diagnosis. Cerebrospinal fluid (CSF) is a clear fluid that surrounds and bathes the brain and spinal cord and may give evidence of myelin breakdown when examined. To obtain a sample of CSF, a fine needle is carefully inserted into the lower back, below the end of the spinal cord as you assume a fetal position and after the area has been numbed. You may feel some pressure, but no pain. After the procedure is done you will be asked to drink fluids, particularly fluids with caffeine to help regenerate the fluid removed, and you should remain lying down for an hour after the procedure and then lie down at home for several hours afterward. You will need someone to drive you home while you lie back in the seat during the trip. The spinal column is very sensitive to being at full pressure, and if you get up before the pressure has returned, you may suffer from a spinal headache that can be quite intense, although it goes away when you lie down again. There is a seventy percent chance that you will be fine the day after the procedure, but you could wake up the morning after with a spinal headache. Should that occur, you will be told to lie down and drink lots of fluid. If the headache is present a second day, you may be sent for what is called a *blood patch*. Blood will be drawn from a vein in your arm, a clot be allowed to form, and that clot will be injected into the area below your spine where the original needle was placed, to close a microscopic leak that presumably occurred and is keeping the spinal column from resuming its normal pressure. I offer this information not to frighten you but rather to let you know that you will not be left with that terrible headache should it occur.

> *I am really a very careful person, so when I went in for a spinal tap I listened carefully to everything the staff there told me. I lay down on the back seat of the car as my wife drove me home after the spinal tap. I drank lots of iced tea and water once back home and rested lying flat on my sofa until bedtime, only getting up carefully to visit the bathroom. I even ate the dinner my wife cooked and brought me almost lying down. The next morning I was up bright and early, sure that I had prevented any chance of a spinal headache. About half an hour later I was hit with the worst headache I could ever imagine. I called the doctor's office and was told that I was part of that unlucky thirty percent of people who got the headache. I was told to go back to bed, drink and lie still, and call the next day if the headache came back. The pain stopped as soon as I lay back down. The next day, about an hour after I got up the pain was back. This time I was told to come in for a blood patch and I returned home pain free and ready to head for work the next day. Fortunately, I won't need another spinal tap.* DAVID

After a lumbar puncture/spinal tap, the CSF is sent to a laboratory for chemical analysis to determine whether there are elevations in immunoglobulin G index and the presence of oligoclonal bands in the CSF that are not present in the serum. At the time of the lumbar puncture/spinal tap a vial of blood is also

What Nurses Know...

Before having a lumbar puncture, you will be asked to sign a consent form. This will give you a chance to talk to your doctor about any concerns you have regarding the need for the procedure, its risks, how it will be done, or what the results will mean.

drawn and submitted to the laboratory for examination. The CSF is usually examined if the MRI is not conclusive but the clinical picture is still suggestive of MS.

More Testing to Diagnose MS

You will be sent to a laboratory where several tubes of blood will be taken from your arm for other lab studies to rule out other causes for your symptoms. Again, it is extremely important to rule out anything else that could be causing your symptoms.

Your health care team wants to make certain that the correct diagnosis is made. You and your family obviously do, too. Because there is no one test to affirm MS, your doctor will decide which of these tests should be done and will discuss with you the rationale for conducting them. We are a society of well-informed and well-educated people. There are always some individuals who are ready to accept the diagnosis their neurologist feels is correct, whereas others want every possible test done before they are ready to accept a diagnosis of a chronic disease such as MS. You are the most important person who will make decisions as to what will be done, and you need to have a comfortable give-and-take relationship with your team of health care professionals.

What Nurses Know ...

Other conditions that can cause symptoms similar to those of MS include vitamin B12 deficiency, folate deficiency, HIV, C-reactive protein, thyroid malfunction, Lyme disease, and rheumatoid arthritis.

Accepted Criteria for a Diagnosis of Multiple Sclerosis

- Symptoms and signs indicating disease of the brain or spinal cord
- Evidence of two or more lesions on the brain from an MRI
- Objective evidence of disease of the brain or spinal cord according to a doctor's exam
- Two or more episodes of symptoms lasting at least twenty-four hours and occurring at least one month apart
- No other explanation for the symptoms

Getting a diagnosis of MS can be a lengthy process. Upon hearing you have MS, you may feel a mixture of emotions, including denial, fear, apprehension, relief, optimism, sadness, and/or hope. For some people the diagnosis can be a relief, but for others it may be shocking. Even when a diagnosis of MS is made, the uncertainty is not over. Because the disease affects no two people the same way, you will no doubt have concerns about the unknown elements of the disease, its course, and its impact on your life. This is completely understandable. We know MS is unpredictable. Sharing your thoughts and emotions with others can help you cope with the diagnosis. Finding a support group run by people from the National Multiple Sclerosis Society (www. nationalmssociety.org) or by a health care professional from your local MS center may be very helpful to you and to your family. Being with other people who have MS and truly understand where you are can make a real difference for you. If, after meeting other individuals who share your diagnosis of MS, you still feel you are struggling, you should not feel embarrassed or different if you need some seek professional help from a counselor to get on the best track.

I am a woman who has always worked so hard to get ahead and do everything right. I was at the top of my class in high school and got a scholarship and job that enabled me to get through college without a huge debt. I found the perfect job with a great company and was really on my way when at age 25 I got the diagnosis of MS. I just couldn't deal with it and was sure that my life was over. I didn't know where to go for help, and I really didn't want any. My doctor insisted that I try a support group, and I finally did go to a meeting. I found people there who understood how I felt and I joined that group. I met Mitch once I decided to come out of my shell, and he wasn't upset that I had MS. He actually came to the support group with me. When Mitch asked me to marry him, I suggested that we talk about MS with the MS nurse at my doctor's office. I wanted to make sure we both understood what we might be in for. I am 36 years old now, and Mitch and I have a five-year-old daughter, Linda, who is perfect. When she was born, we took her in to meet the support group, and they all claimed to be honorary aunts and uncles. I was started on an injectable medication for my MS that I hate to have to take, but I won't miss a dose, because I would hate to look back and think what might have been. My life after my diagnosis with MS didn't end, and we have learned to live, and live well, even though it is still with us. SUSAN

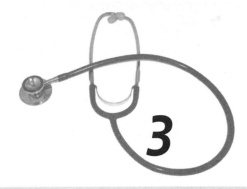

3

Treatments for Multiple Sclerosis

My grandmother's best friend had multiple sclerosis. I remember
visiting her and seeing her in a wheelchair. She said there was
nothing she could take for her disease. Grandmother was so upset
when I got my diagnosis of multiple sclerosis, but I told her that
my doctor said there are medications now that help people with
multiple sclerosis. I'll be learning about them.   ANNA MARIE

Multiple sclerosis (MS) has been with us throughout the ages. It
is certainly not a new disease.

In his book *Multiple Sclerosis: The History of a Disease*,
Dr. T. Jock Murray recounted one of the earliest recorded cases
of MS, that of Saint Lidwina the Virgin, who was born in 1380 in
Schiedam, Holland. After an ice skating accident at age 16, she
had an illness over the next thirty-seven years that had many
features of what we would now identify as MS. Lidwina was later
canonized as the patron saint of figure skating. Murray also

noted that Jean-Martin Characot (1825–1893) is widely considered the first neurologist to put MS on the map as "disseminated sclerosis."

The history of treating MS is interesting but, for those who have had to live with it, developments in treatment have been infuriatingly slow. Compared to other neurological illnesses, such as Alzheimer's disease, however, we have come a very long way in a short time. There is no known cure for MS at this time; there are, however, therapies that may slow the disease. The goal of treatment is to decrease disability, control symptoms, and help you maintain a normal quality of life.

There was no approved drug therapy that could profoundly change the treatment of MS, or alter its course, until 1993, when Betaseron, the first disease-modifying medication, was approved by the U.S. Food and Drug Administration (FDA). Fortunately, Betaseron was followed by the other approved disease-modifying therapies we have today: Avonex, Copaxone, Rebif, Extavia, Tysabri; and, as of September 2010, an oral drug, Gilenya, and Novantrone (an immunosuppressant). All of these drugs decrease the frequency and severity of clinical attacks, decrease the appearance of new symptoms, and slow the rate of disability progression. Betaseron, Avonex, Copaxone, Rebif, Extavia, and Gilenya modulate the immune system, which means that they influence how the immune system functions in the long term.

It is important for you to know about all of the drug therapies that have been approved for MS. If your doctor suggests a medication for you, you will need to know why. In most instances, you will work with your health care team to select the drug therapy that will fit best into your life. The good thing is that all of these medications are becoming more and more user friendly for people with MS, and there are many new drugs currently undergoing research trials. All of the disease-modifying medications discussed in this chapter have been approved by the FDA for treatment of the relapsing forms of MS (i.e., relapsing–remitting and progressive-relapsing; see Chapter 1) as well as secondary progressive MS. They are approved for secondary progressive MS

What Nurses Know...

There are existing drug therapies that can make a difference in MS, and many more are currently being developed. You will need to know about them all, discuss them with your health care team, and make certain that you are receiving the treatment that is best for you.

when the patient continues to experience relapses. Secondary progressive patients may continue to have relapses though they progress between their relapses. The immunotherapies are not approved for secondary progressive patients not experiencing relapses. None are a cure for MS, and they may work differently for different people. None of these medications make a person feel better. They all have side effects that may make you feel worse, although your health care team will work with you to minimize those side effects. You should view these medications as an investment in your future. Managing and treating MS in an ongoing process.

Betaseron

Betaseron was approved by the FDA in 1993. It is known in generic form as *interferon beta-1b* and is made in bacterial cells. Twenty-five milligrams are injected subcutaneously—under the skin—every other day. Betaseron is approved for the treatment of relapsing forms of MS and for treating patients who have experienced a first clinical episode and whose magnetic resonance imaging (MRI) features are consistent with MS. Betaseron can be administered with or without an injector. An injector is a device that will hold a syringe filled with medication. The injector is

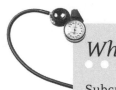

placed on the area to be injected, a button is pressed, and the medication is automatically dispensed. An injector makes it easy for anyone frightened by needles to administer their medication. Including time in clinical trials, there are more than twenty years of clinical experience in using Betaseron.

Betaseron, like all medications, has side effects. Thankfully, there are ways to help you deal with these side effects. Patients can experience flu-like symptoms after their injections, including muscle aches and pains, but not the vomiting and diarrhea one can experience with the flu. By taking acetaminophen (Tylenol), ibuprofen (Motrin), naproxen (Aleve), or aspirin before your injection, and by administering your injection at bedtime, this side effect and be controlled, and it usually lessens over time. You will be instructed as to how to measure the volume or concentration of your Betaseron injections, from an initial low dose to the final, intended dose level so that you become used to the medication and experience fewer side effects. We call this process *titrating* the dose.

Injection site reactions can occur where Betaseron has been injected. Reactions generally include a reddened area of the skin that is not painful and does not itch but certainly isn't attractive. With proper injection techniques this side effect usually lessens over time. What can help is making certain you inject properly; applying a warm, moist compress or washcloth to the area you plan to inject and then applying a cool compress to the area after the injection. Make certain there is no medication on the outside of your needle. It is very important that you vary the sites of your

What Nurses Know...

To titrate means to measure the volume or concentration of your medication so that you begin with a low dose and move to higher doses, giving your body a chance to get used to the medication.

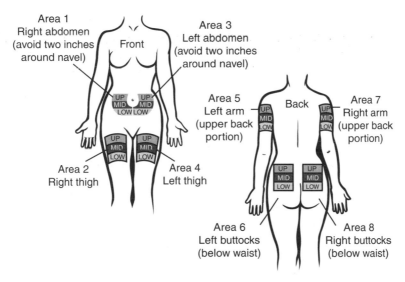

Injection rotation sites for subcutaneous MS interferon injections.

injections. You may use the back of your arms, your stomach, your thighs, and your buttocks (see Figure above).

A prescription for Cordran Tape, to be applied after you inject, can help with site-related reactions. If you find your injections to be painful, your doctor can prescribe a topical anesthetic, such as

What Nurses Know...

Before administering a Betaseron injection, do the following:

1. Wash your hands (anyone else involved also should wash his or her hands).
2. Prepare the area with a prep solution (i.e., rubbing alcohol or other sterilizer) or wash with soap and water.
3. Apply a warm, moist compress to the injection site before injecting.
4. Use a cold compress after injecting if the spot feels painful.
5. Be sure to vary your sites, selecting a new site for each injection.

EMLA cream or a Lidoderm patch. In the event that you develop a reddened area that becomes open or scabs over, call your doctor.

Betaseron has been known to cause liver abnormalities. Your health care practitioner will arrange for you to have your blood levels checked at regular intervals to observe your liver function, make certain that you are not anemic, and ensure that you have normal white blood cell counts and that your thyroid functions are normal. Betaseron is an interferon, and interferons have a reputation of occasionally causing depression, so be sure to report any mood or behavior changes noted by you or your family that could indicate depression. The fact that you have a chronic disease can itself cause you to feel depressed at times, so it is important to be evaluated by a professional.

Betaseron has a support program, BETAPLUS, that employs nurses who work with your doctor to make certain you have the support that you need. A BETA Nurse or a nurse in your local MS center will train you or your significant other to administer your injection. You will be instructed to contact BETA Nurses, who are available 24/7, if you have questions. Once your drug has been prescribed, the staff at BETAPLUS will research your insurance and arrange for you to get the drug. If you have no insurance, or have a copay that you are unable to afford, they will work to make it possible for you to have the drug.

Avonex

The next immunotherapy, Avonex, became available in 1996. Avonex is known in its generic form as *interferon beta-1a* and is prepared in mammalian cells. It is injected via an intramuscular (into the muscle) injection, 30 mcg once each week. It is FDA approved to treat relapsing forms of MS as well as for a first episode if your MRI is consistent with MS. Your prescriber will order 1-inch 25-gauge needles or 1.25-inch 23-gauge needles for you depending on your size and weight.

Again, Avonex is an interferon and thus causes side effects. A major side effect can be flu-like symptoms presenting as muscle aches and pains. The medication should thus be administered at bedtime and can be accompanied by a drug to prevent the symptoms, such as acetaminophen, ibuprofen, aspirin, or naproxen. If you experience flu-like symptoms the next day, take another dose of medication for flu symptoms. Your practitioner may suggest that you titrate your administrations of Avonex over a few weeks until you reach a full dose. The good news is that these side effects usually become less of a problem with time. As with Betaseron, you will be instructed to have regular laboratory tests for anemia and liver abnormalities because Avonex is detoxified or broken down in the liver. You also should be aware that, like Betaseron, Avonex is an interferon and thus can cause depression. Any signs of depression noted by you or your family should be reported to your prescribing physician. Because Avonex is an intramuscular injection you very seldom will have redness at the injection site. If you are giving your own injections, you can learn to inject the medication into your thigh. Your care partner or a family member may give the injection into the deltoid muscle in your arm once trained to do so. Avonex must stored in a refrigerator. It should not be out of the refrigerator for more than twelve hours before you inject, but it should be at room temperature when it is injected. Biogen Idec, that company that manufactures Avonex, employs staff at MS ActiveSource, a Web site for MS patients (www.msactivesource.com), who will accept your prescription, once it has been sent in, and will research your insurance for you (i.e., to see if your insurer will cover the cost). They will let you know where the prescription can be filled and/or arrange for it to be mailed to you. Once you receive your Avonex, you must receive injection training from a nurse at your local MS center or from a nurse at a health care agency contracted by Biogen Idec. Nurses at MS ActiveSource will remain available to answer any of your questions during the hours of 8:00 a.m. to 8:00 p.m. EST.

Copaxone

The next immunotherapy, Copaxone (glatiramer acetate), was introduced in 1996 after receiving FDA approval for the treatment of relapsing-remitting MS as well as for patients who have experienced a first clinical episode and have MRI features consistent with MS. Copaxone is administered every day, 20 mg subcutaneously. Copaxone was developed in Israel many years ago by Teva Neuroscience. It has gone from having to be frozen and then mixed before each injection to being premixed and available in a syringe with a small-bore 29-gauge needle and an injector. Copaxone is not an interferon but rather a substitute antigen that mimics myelin basic protein. It does not cause flu-like symptoms and so may be administered at any time of the day that fits your schedule, although it should be given at the same time each day. I usually suggest to patients that they load the injector at night before bed and give themselves the injection after showering in the morning, when the skin is nice and warm. Of course, you may give yourself the injection before bedtime if you prefer. Copaxone should be stored in the refrigerator but may be left out for a week or more at a time. By loading the injector the night before you can be certain that your drug is at room temperature. Copaxone may be administered without an injector if you prefer. You may experience a light burning sensation after the injection, but it may be so slight that you may not really notice it. If you inject in the morning after your shower, by the time you have finished dressing you won't notice a burning sensation. Again, it is important that you vary injection sites, as shown in the Figure below.

Follow the diagram and rotate injections in your abdomen, the back of your arms, your thighs and your buttocks. We in the field like to call this doing the "macarena."

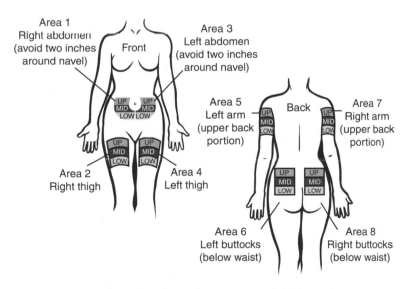

Injection rotation sites for subcutaneous MS interferon injections.

Because Copaxone is not an interferon it is not associated with promoting depression and does not cause injury to the liver. Your health care team will probably order labwork, as would be the procedure if you were not on immunotherapy. The most common side effects of Copaxone are redness, pain, swelling, itching, or a lump at the injection site, all of which are usually mild. You could experience an immediate postinjection reaction that includes flushing of the face, a feeling of tightness in the chest, heart palpitations, anxiety, and shortness of breath that may last up to fifteen minutes. This can be scary, but the reaction is not cardiac or pulmonary in origin. It occurs only sporadically in perhaps ten percent of people taking Copaxone and will probably never occur again. You'll probably feel better if you report the event, should it occur, to your health care provider. Shared Solutions is a resource group for patients on Copaxone sponsored by Teva Neuroscience.. Nurses certified in MS are available for support 24/7. This group arranges with your insurance company for you to get the drug once your prescriber sends them your prescription and can arrange for in-home injection training unless you are to receive training at your local MS center. They can also offer referrals for sources of financial assistance if necessary.

Rebif

Rebif (interferon beta-1a) was made available for the treatment of MS after being approved by the FDA in 2002. Rebif is given three times a week: either Monday, Wednesday, and Friday or Tuesday, Thursday, and Saturday. Like the other drugs discussed thus far, Rebif is injected subcutaneously, 44 mcg per injection. Rebif is indicated for the treatment of relapsing forms of MS. The side effects you may experience from Rebif are much like those associated with Betaseron or Avonex. There may be mild flu-like symptoms and redness at the injection site. Titrating the injections over the first month to the final 44-mcg dose lessens those side effects. Rebif is stored in the refrigerator but is safe outside the refrigerator for a month and should be injected at room temperature. You will be told that side effects diminish when your drug is injected at bedtime into a site that has been warmed by a warm, moist washcloth. EMLA cream or Lidoderm patches may be prescribed for you if you find the injection to be painful, although that is not a frequent problem. Cordran Tape may help if you have red injection sites. It is very important that you follow instructions for the "macarena" using all of the approved sites shown again in the Figure below.

You will be doing injections in your abdomen, the back of your arms, your thighs, and buttocks. If you have a red site that develops a scab, you should contact your doctor. Rebif has an injector to make giving the injections more user friendly and is administered via a 29-gauge needle. Most people elect to use the injector, but you can be instructed to give the injection without the injector should you prefer. You should have regular labs drawn to test for liver abnormalities, evaluate thyroid functions, and discern low red or white blood counts. MS LifeLines (www.mslifelines.com) is a Rebif resource, sponsored by EMD Serono and Pfizer, manufacturers of Rebif, whose staff will process

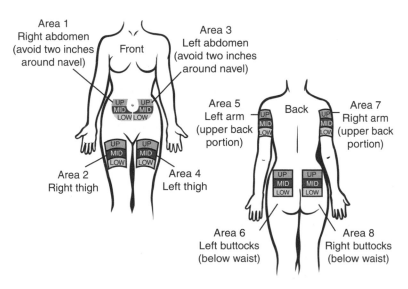

Injection rotation sites for subcutaneous MS interferon injections.

your prescription when sent to them by your prescriber, verify that your insurance plan covers the drug, and arrange for you to receive your drug in the most convenient way. They also will help you with financial assistance and provide additional support. Nurses certified in MS are available through MS LifeLines to answer questions from 8:00 a.m. through 8:00 p.m. EST. MS Lifelines also offers training in Rebif administration by an MS nurse, or you can be trained at your local MS center.

Extavia

Extavia (interferon beta-1b) was made available after receiving FDA approval in 2009. Extavia is the exact same formulation as Betaseron and is manufactured on the very same manufacturing line as Betaseron, although it is marketed by a different pharmaceutical company. It is available to administer with a 27-gauge needle and a user-friendly injector. It is approved for the treatment of relapsing forms of MS and secondary progressive MS with relapses and for individuals who have experienced a first clinical episode and have MRI features consistent with MS. The side effects of Extavia mirror those of Betaseron. It is injected subcutaneously in increments of 25 mg. You will be instructed to titrate the drug when beginning its use to minimize side effects. It should be administered at bedtime on warm, moist skin, rotating sites used for injection as depicted in the Figure on the following page.

Regular labs will be ordered by your doctor to monitor thyroid function, liver function, and blood counts. As with the other interferons, you should be aware of potential depression, and be sure to report any signs you might recognize as depression. As with Betaseron, you need to be faithful at rotating injection sites, using your abdomen, highs, backs of your arms, and your buttocks. Novartis, the company that markets Extavia, provides the Extavia Patient Support Program (www.extavia.com) that can act as your support system as soon as your prescription is submitted by your prescriber. Reimbursement support and nursing support

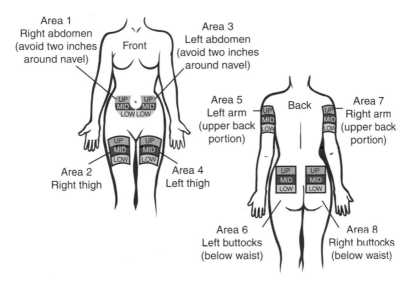

Area 1
Right abdomen
(avoid two inches
around navel)

Front

Area 3
Left abdomen
(avoid two inches
around navel)

Area 5
Left arm
(upper back
portion)

Back

Area 7
Right arm
(upper back
portion)

Area 2
Right thigh

Area 4
Left thigh

Area 6
Left buttocks
(below waist)

Area 8
Right buttocks
(below waist)

Injection rotation sites for subcutaneous MS interferon injections.

are available from 8:00 a.m. until 8:00 p.m. EST. The program also offers specialty pharmacy support and drug delivery and a copay assistance program, as well as injection instruction in your home.

I have multiple sclerosis, and when I was diagnosed my doctor was so excited to be able to tell me that he could prescribe a medication for me that could help prevent or decrease the intensity of flares of my disease and could prevent disability. I was excited about that as well until I learned that any of the drugs he might prescribe I would have to inject. I knew I didn't want to give injections, but I agreed to go ahead and give it a try. I was really good at injecting for about four months and then it got to me. I decided to give myself a "holiday" for just a week. It was great not injecting…no red spots. I just forgot to go back! Six months later I had what we all termed a "real exacerbation." My girlfriend

What Nurses Know...

Betaseron, Avonex, Copaxone, Rebif, and Extavia are all drugs that need to be injected. They WILL NOT help you if they are left in the refrigerator or on the shelf and not taken as you have been directed to take them! They don't make you feel better a the time they are taken. If you skip a dose, it is easy to skip the next one, and the drug can't make a difference if you don't take it.

took me to the emergency room because I couldn't walk. I was treated with IV steroids, and I am better now, but you can bet that I am back on my injections and don't plan any more holidays. KEVIN

Tysabri

Tysabri (natalizumab) is also an immune-modulating drug, but it is delivered by infusion (into a vein), and this is done in an infusion facility. Tysabri gained final approval in 2006 from the FDA for the treatment of relapsing forms of MS as a monotherapy (i.e., not used in combination with any other disease-modifying medication). It is infused as 300 mg intravenously every four weeks. It is recommended for people who have had inadequate response to other medications or who are not able to tolerate another disease-modifying therapy.

Tysabri is produced in a laboratory and is a monoclonal antibody that attaches to a specific surface structure of the immune T cells. It slows the T cells from moving out of the bloodstream and into the brain and spinal cord where they may stimulate inflammation that can result in MS attacks. People who take

Tysabri are at increased risk for a rare and generally fatal brain disease called *progressive multifocal leukoencephalopathy* (PML). There are no interventions known at this time to cure PML once it occurs. There were three cases of PML in clinical trials in patients who were also taking another immunomodulating or immunosuppressing medication. Other cases have been reported in the postmarketing phase. Researchers have not yet been able to precisely estimate the absolute risk of PML for patients taking Tysabri. The newest figure is that 1.71 persons per 1,000 who are on the drug for two years or longer will develop PML.

Physicians who prescribe Tysabri, and patients who take the drug, as well as infusion centers where the drug is administered, must enroll in a mandatory registry program, called the TOUCH Prescribing Program, which provides constant monitoring for any signs that might suggest PML. Tysabri is not recommended to be used by anyone whose immune system is weakened by disease or by drugs that alter the immune system, and it must be used as monotherapy; that is, it may not be used with other disease-modifying therapies. Again, at this time we do not know everything about the safety of long-term use of Tysabri. Other side effects of Tysabri are headaches; fatigue; urinary tract infections; depression; lower respiratory infections; joint pain; chest discomfort; liver abnormalities; and allergic or hypersensitivity reactions within two hours of infusion, seen as dizziness, fever, rash, nausea, low blood pressure, and difficulty breathing. Tysabri does have a reimbursement program that will work with your insurance company to cover the drug as well as a copay assistance program and a program for individuals without insurance. The Tysabri Mentor Program (www.tysabri.com) employs nurses who provide educational support for users.

Gilenya

Gilenya (fingolimod) is the first orally administered drug approved for the treatment of people with relapsing forms of MS to reduce the frequency of clinical exacerbations and to delay the accumulation of physical disability. It was approved by the FDA in September 2010. It is ingested as 0.5 mg once daily and may be taken with or without food. It is a capsule and comes in a blister pack.

Gilenya is the newest drug for MS in the market, and it comes with important safety information. It may have serious side effects. It may cause your heart rate to slow down, especially after your first dose, with the heart usually slowing down the most about six hours after you take that first dose. If your heart rate does slow down, you might feel dizzy or tired or be aware of a slow or irregular heartbeat. Your doctor will arrange for you to be observed for the first six hours after you take your first dose to see if you have any serious side effects. Your slow heart rate will usually return to normal within one month after you start taking Gilenya. If you have a history of heart problems, your doctor may suggest that Gilenya is not the treatment for you.

Gilenya lowers the number of white blood cells in your blood and can increase your risk of serious infections. Call your doctor immediately if you have symptoms of an infection, such as fever, tiredness, body aches, chills, or nausea or vomiting while taking Gilenya.

Gilenya has been known to cause a vision problem called *macular edema.* Macular edema can cause some of the same vision symptoms as an MS attack of optic neuritis (inflammation of the optic nerve fibers; see Chapter 4), but with macular edema you may not notice any symptoms. It usually starts in the first three to four months after you start taking Gilenya. Your doctor should arrange for your vision to be tested before you start taking Gilenya and then again three to four months after you start or at any time you notice vision changes during your treatment with Gilenya. Your risk of macular edema may be higher if you are diabetic. You will be instructed to call your doctor if you have blurriness or shadows in the center of your vision, a blind spot in the center of your vision, sensitivity to light, or unusually tinted vision.

Elevations of liver function tests may occur in patients who are taking Gilenya, so you will be instructed to have regular laboratory testing. There are no adequate studies of Gilenya in

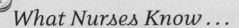

What Nurses Know...

You need always to tell your doctor about all of your medical conditions, as well as any medications, vitamins, herbal remedies, and so on, that you are taking, before starting any new drugs.

pregnant women, so you should not become pregnant while on the drug or for at least two months following its discontinuation. If you should become pregnant while on Gilenya, contact your doctor at once.

You need always to tell your doctor about all of your medical conditions before you start taking any drugs. Before starting Gilenya you need to report whether you have an irregular or abnormal heartbeat, a heart rate of fewer than fifty-five beats a minute, any heart problems or history of fainting, any eye problems, diabetes, any breathing problems, any liver problems, or high blood pressure. You need to let your doctor know if you have ever had chicken pox or if you have received the vaccine for chicken pox. Your doctor may do a blood test for chicken pox virus, and you may need to get the vaccine for chicken pox and then wait one month before you start taking Gilenya. The most common side effects of Gilenya include headache, flu, diarrhea, back pain, abnormal liver tests, and a cough. Gilenya, made by Novartis, has a patient support system that will work with your insurance company to see to it that you get the drug as soon as your prescriber submits your prescription. The Gilyena Support Program Call Center is available by phone 8:00 a.m.–9:00 p.m. ET, Monday through Friday at 1-877-408-4974. The support program staff will work with you to provide copay assistance, if needed. They also provide assistance to people with no insurance and will provide help in regard to some of the testing you need when

What Nurses Know...

The convenience of oral therapy needs to be balanced against other factors, such as safety. Gilenya has been shown to be safe in studies to date, but these studies have been only one to two years in length. The injectable therapies have had much larger exposure, in some cases more than fifteen to twenty years. Side effects that arise after years of exposure may not be revealed until larger number of people have taken the drug.

starting Gilenya. A Nurse Navigator is available to help answer your questions about Gilenya 24 hours a day, 7 days a week for urgent needs at 1-877-408-4974.

People who are already taking a disease-modifying drug therapy will need to consider the effectiveness of their current drug therapy and, if they are doing well, will need to decide whether it is better to continue with a successful treatment or to switch to a treatment that may or may not be as effective for them and may carry with it different side effects. Newly diagnosed people will need to consult their health care provider to discuss the efficacy and known safety of all available medications and make an informed decision as to what they want to take.

Novantrone

The last FDA-approved drug for the treatment of MS at this time is an immunosuppressant (i.e., a drug that suppresses the immune system) called Novantrone (mitoxantrone). Novantrone was approved by the FDA in 2000 and was originally developed to treat certain forms of cancer. It was approved for use in MS for worsening cases of relapsing-remitting MS as well as for progressive-relapsing MS or secondary progressive MS. It is generally reserved for people with MS whose disease is seriously worsening.

Novantrone is given by intervenous infusion in a medical facility in eight to twelve lifetime doses over a two- to three-year period, usually at three-month intervals. The total lifetime dose is limited in order to avoid possible heart damage. People taking Novantrone are required to have tests of heart function—an echocardiogram or electrocardiogram—before each dose. It cannot be given to people with preexisting heart problems or people with liver disease or certain blood disorders. It cannot be given to women who may be pregnant or may become pregnant; thus, pregnancy testing for pre-menopausal women., Regular blood testing and screening for possible urinary tract infections, is required before each infusion. It can cause blue-green urine twenty-four hours after infusion and lowers the white blood cell count, heightening the patient's risk for infections. The drug can

What Nurses Know...

How do you know if you are taking the right medication? Ask yourself the following questions.

1. *Are you tolerating the medication?*
2. *Are you having more relapses, or have your relapses decreased?*
3. *How are your symptoms?*
4. *What does your MRI look like?*

Share all of this information with your health care team. Drug therapy is a complex issue, and it takes someone who really knows you and really knows everything that's available for MS to help walk you through it.

also cause bone marrow suppression with fatigue and bruising as well as nausea; hair thinning; bladder infections; liver damage; and acute myelogenous leukemia, a type of cancer. Cancer and heart problems may develop in people who are on Novantrone therapy. People considering Novantrone for worsening MS need to include members of their family support system in counseling with their prescriber before making any decision start the drug.

All Immunotherapies

All of the medications available at this time can change the course of MS. If you note the FDA approval dates of the immunotherapies discussed thus far, you can see that the injectable therapies have been available and used now for a long time, up to fifteen to twenty years. These medications, although they are not cures, have made a big difference in the lives of people with MS.

> *My wife has had MS for the past 40 years. At first, she had very few symptoms and got around with no problem. Gradually, she became disabled and for the past ten years has needed total care. I go to MS programs and learn about the therapies that are available today, and I so wish they had been available for my Debbie. Maybe she would be walking today. I am glad they will make a difference for people diagnosed today.* JOHN

There are more drugs in the pipeline at this time; some of them will be available soon. Some will be in pill form, and some will be in IV form. This is an exciting time for all who work in the field of MS and certainly for those who live with the disease. Health care professionals will be examining the efficacy of these drugs, looking hard at their safety data, and making careful informed decisions before deciding to use them. Some of you will be first in line to try new medications as they are released. Others will want to wait and see. All of you will want to learn all that you can about new drugs for MS and watch for new drugs as they come

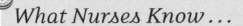

What Nurses Know...

There is no one specific drug that's better for everyone, no one "best" drug. Everyone is different, and everyone's disease is different. It is very important to work with your health care provider to find the drug that works best for you.

on the market. Watch for information as it becomes available for laquinimod, cladrabine, teriflunomide, dimethyl fumarate, alemtuzumab, rituximab, and daclizumab, all of which are in clinical trials, along with other drugs. Be aware that these are generic names that will probably differ from the names assigned if and when these drugs are marketed.

While researching MS, you may have come across a condition called *chronic cerebro-spinal venous insufficiency*, which is an abnormality in blood drainage from the brain and spinal cord that may contribute to nervous system damage in MS, a hypothesis first proposed by Dr. Paulo Zambori in Italy. He studied sixty-five patients and proposed treating them through an endovascular surgical procedure. He has recommended larger studies, and MS societies in the United States and Canada in conjunction with other associations around the world, will coordinate information and share research data on this procedure (www.nationalmssociety.org). This remains yet another thing for you to watch.

Your health care provider will work with you to help make decisions regarding the treatment you want. You need to know that the MS health care community will be there to support the decisions you make. Remember, the most important thing about selecting a medication that will slow the natural course of MS is to adhere to that medication's dosing procedures and schedule. Nothing can help if you don't commit to taking it regularly and as directed.

Many people think they cannot learn to give themselves injections. All people can learn to inject a medication, no matter how difficult they think it will be at first. For people with deeply held fears relating to needle use, techniques such as visualization, deep breathing, and other management tools can be implemented by nurses or psychologists. Again, you must always administer your drugs as prescribed. The injection schedule differs according to the drug selected, but none of the medications will make a difference for you if they are left on the shelf or in the refrigerator and not taken. There will be lots of times when you think that you just cannot inject again. You don't feel better after your injections. Many times, you feel worse. If you truly can't tolerate your injections and find yourself taking long holidays from using them because of your anxiety, you may want to look into an oral drug therapy. Oral medications may seem easier, but we all know that it is easy to forget and skip a pill. What you must do is view your medication as an investment in your future. This is something you can do for yourself that can make a positive difference in your life.

My friend Ginger and I both have MS. We go to the same MS center and met in the waiting room when we had appointments on the same day. Ginger is "textbook." She remains on the medication she started six years ago and is doing so well. I, on the other hand, am not "textbook." I have been on everything! I have had flu-like symptoms that sent me to bed and site reactions that make me a charter member of the red spot club. As if that isn't enough, I continue to have regular flare-ups—not serious instances, but I have them. I even had a bad reaction when I tried Tysabri. I have an appointment to talk with my doctor about Gilenya now that it is available. I think I am the perfect candidate for an oral drug, and I am keeping my fingers crossed that this will be with answer for me. FLORRIE

Many medications are used off label for MS (i.e., used to treat MS even though the FDA approved the drug for a different

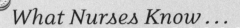

What Nurses Know . . .

I like to suggest that you look to someone in your family or a special friend as a support system and ask that person to help you if you choose an injectable medication. That help can take the form of moral support, of setting timers to remind you to do your injections, or of helping you with the actual injecting. Should you decide on an oral medication, that person can help remind you to take the pill.

purpose). We don't have "the cure," and MS is a progressive disease, so when a person's MS continues to progress while taking approved medications, health care professionals often look for that "something else" that might be an add-on medication or used by itself. Most of the drugs used like this are immunosuppressive drugs. Infusions of low-dose Cytoxan (cyclophosphamide), and oral drugs approved for rheumatoid arthritis, such as methotrexate (e.g., Rheumatrex, Trexall) or Imuran (azthioprine), may be used off label for MS. Some people improve with intravenous immunoglobulin at monthly intervals. Your doctor will discuss the pros and cons of these medications with you as well as their side effects if he or she feels they should be considered in your treatment.

Most people with MS experience exacerbations, or attacks or flares which often last from one to three months. Acute symptoms must be present for at least twenty-four to forty-eight hours, without any signs of infection or fever, before the treating physician may consider it to be a true relapse. Steroids are used to treat these individual exacerbations or relapses and sometimes are given in monthly or bimonthly intervals to prevent the progression of your MS. Steroids can be those taken orally, such as prednisone or Decadron (dexamethasone); intravenously, such as Solu-Medrol (methylprednisolone); or by injection, such as Acthar Gel (corticotropin).

All steroids are usually given for three to five days. I discuss the use of steroids in detail in Chapter 4. Long-term use of steroids is not generally recommended. They can cause many side effects when given over a long period of time and may have no effect on the long-term progression of MS.

There are a variety of symptoms that health care professionals treat specifically. These treatments work, although they do nothing to stop the progression of the disease. Symptoms that can often be controlled or relieved with medicine include

- Fatigue
- Muscle stiffness, spasticity, and tremors
- Urinary problems and constipation
- Pain and abnormal sensations
- Depression
- Sexual difficulties

These are discussed in Chapter 4 as well.

Advice Regarding All Medications

Work with your support nurses in your local MS center or those employed by the support system provided by the manufacturer of your drug. If you are injecting your drug, check to make certain that your technique is correct. With subcutaneous injections you may experience membership in the "red spot club" early on. You may have some red areas after you inject with any of the drugs. Usually the red areas last only a few hours, although in some instances they may be there for several days. They almost always diminish with long term use of your drug.

If areas of redness are a problem, talk with your support staff. They can come up with lots of "tricks" that help. I have mentioned some of those in my descriptions of the medications this chapter, but the "tricks" can be suited to your needs. If you find you cannot tolerate a medication, you can change to another. After long-term use all of the injectable drugs given subcutaneously can cause *induration*, a condition in which you can see a dip in your skin in the area where you have injected. This is seen most often with Copaxone, but it can occur with any of the subcutaneous injections. To prevent this, the most important thing you can do is that "macarena" move to vary your injection sites, and be sure not inject in the same place over and over again. Your support nurse can help you find new sites to inject if necessary.

None of the drugs discussed in this chapter have been approved for use during pregnancy. If you are planning a pregnancy, you will need to talk with your health care provider and decide whether and when to come off your medication. If you find that you are pregnant, contact your prescriber at once.

I worked with people with MS for many, many years, long before we had medications that could change the course of the disease. For years, my colleagues and I could only manage symptoms. I have seen the difference in care and the impact that these drugs have had on people living with MS. Until there is a cure for MS there will always be some symptoms to manage, but these drugs can make a real difference in your ability to enjoy the quality of life you find acceptable.

Reference

Murray, T. J. (2005). *Multiple sclerosis: The history of a disease.* New York: Demos Medical Publishing.

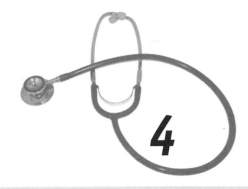

4

Multiple Sclerosis Symptoms and How We Treat Them

I am faithful at taking my immunotherapy and still I experience some multiple sclerosis (MS) symptoms. I think they come to remind me that I do have MS. I have learned that I may discuss my symptoms with my MS support staff and that they are there to suggest treatments. I have MS and I am going to experience some symptoms, but I don't have to suffer in silence.   MARY JEAN

Multiple sclerosis (MS) directly affects the central nervous system (CNS), which comprises the brain and the spinal cord. All of the components of the CNS communicate with each other, although different areas of the brain and spinal cord are responsible for different kinds of movements and sensations. MS symptoms depend on the location of the area of sclerosis or scarring, or what we refer to as *lesions*. Lesions vary from one individual to another, so no two persons with MS have exactly the same symptoms, and no two cases of MS are exactly alike. Symptoms vary from one person to another and may be in the form of mild disturbances in one person or moderate or more severe disturbances in another. Symptoms may appear as an acute attack, termed an *exacerbation* or *relapse or a flare*, or they may become more chronic, with ensuing clinical or functional deterioration.

It is natural when you are diagnosed with MS to think that anything that happens to you is probably a symptom of MS. If you have an MS diagnosis, then any symptom you have must be due to MS! I have had patients call me complaining of a runny nose, sneezing, and a sore throat wanting to know if these are MS symptoms. My answer is that it sounds as though these are symptoms of a cold but to take good care of yourself and always feel free to call and check on problems that you feel might be due to MS. In this chapter, I examine symptoms typical of MS. When you experience symptoms that may be exacerbations of your MS, you will need help to decide if they are serious enough to be considered an exacerbation or relapse (see Chapter 5 for a more detailed discussion of exacerbations/relapses). You will need to talk with the doctor's office or MS nurse to determine if your symptoms need to be treated as symptoms or if you are having an exacerbation or relapse that needs special treatment.

In the sections that follow, I address common MS symptoms, including fatigue; depression; weakness; vision changes; bowel and bladder dysfunction; sexual problems; spasticity; sensory

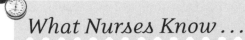

symptoms, such as numbness and tingling; pain; and cognitive changes. Less common symptoms include tremor and speech disturbances, swallowing problems, and vertigo. The important thing for you to remember is that MS symptoms can be treated: You should not feel that you need to "grin and bear it."

Fatigue

I had such a time with fatigue that it became a real family problem. My husband was certain that he knew all about "being tired." He said all I needed was to get a good night's sleep. I didn't need to cop out on things! I mentioned this to my MS nurse, and she scheduled a time for my husband to come with me to see her and talk about my MS fatigue. My husband listened! He is there to help and understand. We know now how to communicate, and it makes such a difference now for us both.   MARLA

Fatigue is considered one of the most, if not *the* most, common causes of disability in MS. It is a subjective lack of physical or mental energy that is perceived to interfere with usual and desired activities, a feeling of physical tiredness or a lack of energy. It comes on easily, without warning, and can appear early in the disease. It is not related to the amount of disability a person may have. More than half of people with MS say that fatigue is their greatest problem. It may appear as an acute problem, a sluggishness that is activity limiting, or it may be a chronic and persistent problem lasting more than six weeks. It limits functional ability and certainly affects quality of life. MS fatigue is thought to be caused by demyelination and axonal damage. It may signal the beginning of an exacerbation, or it might be the presenting symptom that brought on the diagnosis of MS. MS fatigue is something that is very difficult for persons who do not have MS to understand, particularly when they are family members. One of my patients once described it as his sitting in a chair with the television on and wanting to change the channel but not having the strength to get up and get the remote to do that. It is not sleepiness but rather a feeling of being completely wiped out.

It is important to understand that there are many causes for, and kinds of, fatigue that people with MS experience. Heat can be one cause of fatigue; cooling equipment, such as cooling vests or cooling scarves, even a cold drink, such as a Slurpee from a 7-Eleven, can control heat-related fatigue. One

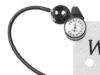

What Nurses Know...

Wearing a cooling scarf that will complement your outfit can be a way to get your body temperature down and alleviate some of your fatigue. You can find them for sale by searching "cooling scarf" on the Internet.

helpful technique is to try wearing no socks to bring your body temperature down.

Lack of sleep causes fatigue, and sleep deprivation can occur when one is stressed, when one doesn't go to bed, when sleep is interrupted by the need to get up because of urinary problems or restless legs, or when one is not able to plan for and get the amount of sleep his or her body requires. Fatigue also can be caused by depression.

When you complain of fatigue, it is very important to work with your health care team to determine the cause of that fatigue. I remember treating a young mother who complained of fatigue. When asked to describe her day, it went something like this: "I get up at 5:30 in the morning to prepare breakfast and school lunches for my three older children, ages 6, 9, and 12. Then I get them off to their school buses and get my 2-year-old off to his day care. I am at work by 8:30. I teach high school English. I am able to leave school by 3:30 to pick up the 2-year-old and get the other children off to soccer and swimming and baseball practice. I am a Girl Scout leader for our 9-year-old. I prepare dinner, oversee homework and baths and bedtime, and then correct papers and prepare lessons for my school students. I am pretty late getting to bed. Then there is laundry and housework on the weekend. My MS really makes me tired!"

What Nurses Know . . .

Fatigue is a real problem with MS. It can be caused by demyelination, but there are other causes as well, so it needs to be carefully evaluated.

I had to explain to this woman that just going over her day made me exhausted! We worked together on ways to accomplish the events of her day using energy conservation techniques. Her husband stepped in to help with dinner and food shopping. The children were made to understand that they had to help by making school lunches and doing laundry. She was able to trade driving assignments for after-school activities with other parents, and by limiting extra expenses such as fast food dinners the family was able to hire a cleaning service to come every other week to free up time on weekends. This gal was able to understand that her fatigue problem was a lifestyle problem probably not due to her MS.

Other illnesses can be the cause of fatigue as well and need to be ruled out. Conditions such as anemia, liver disease, thyroid disease, infections, and pain need to be checked as possible reasons for fatigue.

There are treatments that can help MS fatigue. One option is medication. One of the medications used to treat MS fatigue is amantadine. Many of the medications used in the treatment of MS are used "off label," that is, they received Food and Drug Administration approval for other medical problems. Amantadine

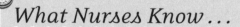

What Nurses Know...

Modafinil (brand names: Provigil, Alertec, Modavigil, Modalert, Modiodal, Modafinilo, Carim, and Vigia) is used to treat excessive sleepiness caused by narcolepsy. Modafinil is in a class of medications called wakefulness-promoting agents. *It works by changing the amounts of certain natural substances in the area of the brain that control sleep and wakefulness. Modafinil may be habit forming. Do not take a larger dose, take it more often, or take it for a longer period of time than prescribed by your doctor.*

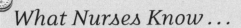

What Nurses Know...

Just six months of yoga significantly reduces fatigue in people with MS according to an Oregon Health & Science University study published in the journal Neurology (Oken BS, Kishiyama MA, Zajdel D. et al, 2010).

is one of these medications. It has been used in Parkinson's disease and to prevent influenza, and it can help some people experiencing MS fatigue. Another medication used off label is Modafinil, which is a drug intended for somnolence—daytime sleepiness—and has been very helpful in treating MS fatigue.

Antidepressants such as Prozac (fluoxetine) are sometimes prescribed for MS fatigue. Nonmedical treatments can also be used to help fatigue. Short "veg out" sessions or rest periods fitted into the day just before the time when fatigue regularly occurs can ward off the fatigue. Take fifteen minutes off a lunch period and use that time later in the workday when you need it, or come home from work and relax for fifteen minutes before starting dinner. Regular exercise is important for persons with MS and actually helps to decrease fatigue. It is important to vary your exercise program when you have MS. Muscle fatigue worsens if one muscle group is repeatedly asked to perform, so an exercise program needs to contain variety.

Depression

I was so upset when I was diagnosed with MS that all I wanted to do was to lie around and cry. I refused to do anything at all. I didn't want to take an antidepressant. I don't like to depend on medications. My doctor talked me into taking an antidepressant just as a trial, and I felt so much better. Now, a year later, I don't need my antidepressant and I am living like I did before MS. JOYCE

Depression is a term that is applied to a wide variety of mood disorders in MS and is common during the course of the disease. Approximately fifty percent of people with MS experience depression at some point during the course of their MS (Patten SB. (2009). Depression may occur at any time, even when things are going well. Depression is a term that is applied to a wide variety of mood disorders in MS. Evidence suggests that it may be a result of the disease process, perhaps due to brain lesions in specific areas that increase the risk of depression. The suicide rate is higher in the MS population than in the general (i.e., healthy) population (Kalb RC, 2008). According to the journal *Neurology*, "Suicidal intent, a potential harbinger for suicide, is common in MS and is strongly associated with major depression, alcohol abuse, and social isolation."

Depression is nothing to be ashamed of and is never your fault. It can be actually a symptom of MS and is caused by complex physical, chemical, and/or emotional processes and drug interactions that medical professionals still do not understand fully. The good news is that, in the hands of the right doctor, depression is treatable.

People with MS and their family members need to be aware of signs of depression, which include the following:

- Feeling sad or empty
- Irritability, crying, or not sleeping well
- Complaints of being tired all day
- Not eating or increased appetite
- Being anxious
- Not wanting to go out with friends
- Loss of interest or pleasure in most activities
- Decreased sex drive
- A feeling of not being able to deal with MS symptoms any more

If you are experiencing any of these symptoms, report them to your doctor, who will review any medications you are taking that may contribute to depression, go over symptoms, perhaps prescribe medications to help with depression, and/or recommend counseling or psychotherapy. He or she will monitor your response to these interventions at regular intervals. Depression can be managed and certainly does not have to be a constant problem. Some of the medications prescribed for MS depression are Prozac (fluoxetine), Zoloft (sertraline), Paxil (paroxetine), Celexa (citalopram), Lexapro (escitalopram), Effexor (venlafaxine), Wellbutrin (bupropion), Cymbalta (duloxetine), Elavil (amitriptyline), Desyrel (trazodone), and Pamelor (nortriptyline). Your doctor will help to find something that can help you.

Bladder Function

I think the thing about my MS that bothers me most is always having to find a bathroom. The first thing I do when I go anywhere is to make certain I know the location of the bathroom. I know this is a common problem for those of us with MS because wherever I go to an MS program, the speaker begins by telling the location of the bathrooms.   EMMA

Problems with bladder function are common in people with MS. Approximately eighty percent of people with MS complain of bladder problems that may vary from annoying to severe (Kalb RC, 2008). Urinary frequency can be such a problem that I learned long ago that if I wanted to know where to find the best restrooms at a nearby shopping mall, I should ask someone with MS. At a support group meeting I once led, the participants readily rated the bathrooms at all businesses at the local malls. Again, this is not something to be embarrassed about. It important to seek treatment right away and not try to hide the problem. There are many excellent treatment options available for bladder function issues. Your treatment provider may describe behavioral and dietary approaches that can reduce your symptoms. A referral to a physical therapist is a great idea, too. Urinary problems are common in MS and very often are easily treated, but if left untreated they can lead to serious problems.

Lesions in the brain and spinal cord are the cause of bladder problems. Symptoms include

- A feeling of urgency and the need to reach the bathroom immediately because of an inability to hold urine
- Frequency
- Having to urinate small amounts very frequently
- Dribbling
- Leaking small amounts of urine
- Hesitancy or difficulty beginning to urinate after the urge to void is felt
- Incontinence is an inability to hold urine in the bladder

The bladder has a capacity to hold 500 milliliters of urine. Normally one experiences an urge to void when the bladder is holding 200 to 300 milliliters. The most common problem in MS is a decreased ability to store urine. Voiding becomes a reflex action, with uninhibited contractions; in these cases we say

What Nurses Know ...

You need to remember that caffeine, aspartame (a sweetener often found in diet soft drinks), and alcohol all increase your need to void frequently.

that one has a small, *spastic* bladder that is causing increased frequency, urgency, dribbling, and/or incontinence. Treatment for this problem would be frequent bathroom breaks with quick access to bathrooms and the use of pads or protective undergarments. If you are experiencing difficulties voiding, decrease your use of bladder irritants such as caffeine, aspartame, and alcohol. Your doctor may prescribe medications called *anticholinergics* such as Detrol LA (talterodine tartrate), Ditropan XL (oxybutynin chloride), Oxytrol (oxybutynin transdermal), Sanctura (trospium), VESIcare (solifenacin), or Enablex (darifenacin).

Another problem can be an inability to empty the bladder. Messages can't be transmitted to or from either the brain or the bladder, and so the bladder becomes large and flaccid. It fills and overfills and causes symptoms of frequency, urgency, dribbling, and incontinence. Treatment involves structured and timed voiding and often-intermittent catheterization to empty the bladder.

As if it were not enough to have either a problem of failure to fill or failure to empty, one can also have a combined dysfunction, called a *conflicting bladder*, whereby the bladder wall contracts while the sphincter remains closed, resulting in urgency followed by hesitancy (difficulty beginning to urinate after the urge to void is felt), or the bladder wall relaxes while the sphincter remains open, resulting in dribbling or incontinence. This problem is usually diagnosed by your health care provider, who

What Nurses Know . . .

Drink fluids all at once, because if you sip, sip, sip, you will feel the urge to go often. Limiting fluid intake is harmful.

can refer you to a urologist, who will do urodynamic testing and determine a treatment regimen.

Try to void about one and a half hours after you drink, stop drinking fluids about two hours before bedtime, and void right before bedtime, but don't limit fluid intake throughout the day or you may cause problems such as constipation. Your body needs water.

Urinary tract infections (UTIs) are frequently seen in people with MS. They are not a direct result of demyelination but occur as a result of retention of urine in the bladder. Certainly, a large, flaccid bladder provides the perfect opportunity for bacteria to grow. When you retain urine, when there is an incomplete emptying of the bladder, not enough fluid intake to flush the bladder, or improper wiping after a bowel movement, a UTI results. A UTI is diagnosed by a urine culture and is easily treated with antibiotics. Symptoms of UTI include frequent urination, urgency, burning or discomfort, and sometimes foul-smelling urine or the presence of blood in the urine. Usually these symptoms occur suddenly, and they may be accompanied by fever. An infection such as a UTI can cause an exacerbation or relapse in MS. When you call your doctor's office or MS nurse to report what you think might be a relapse, you will often be asked questions to rule out a UTI.

Bowel Problems

I was really tired of having to find a bathroom all the time, so I decided to cut out liquids. There were no eight glasses of water for me anymore, and I even started eating my meals with nothing to drink alongside. I put aside the bottle of water I used to keep next to my bed. Then I began to experience constipation. That was the last straw! I confessed to my MS nurse my new problem, and she helped me return liquids to my diet along with adding fiber. I am back to normal again.　KIMBERLY

Bowel problems are less frequent than bladder problems. The main problems seen are constipation and, less often, incontinence. Constipation can becomes a problem if one is experiencing bladder problems and decides to limit fluid intake. Water that the body needs is absorbed as the stool passes through the colon, and the stool becomes hard and difficult to pass. Weakness and fatigue may limit physical activity, which slows bowel activity, and the stool moves more slowly through the colon so that more water is absorbed, making constipation worse. Demyelination can again be the cause, interfering with nerve transmission necessary for normal defecation. Medications taken for other problems also may cause constipation.

Diet is very important in maintaining proper bowel function. It is important to drink adequate amounts of fluid and have a diet that includes adequate amounts of fiber. Food items that are high in fiber include

- Raw fruits and vegetables
- Whole grain breads
- Legumes
- Nuts
- Seeds
- Cereals
- Grains some pastas

Various online sites list food fiber counts. Develop a bowel program consisting of a time when you can relax and have time in the bathroom. It is often helpful to do this after a relaxing

What Nurses Know ...

You need to have the same frequency of bowel movements that you had before your diagnosis of MS. Going three to four days without a bowel movement is too long!

cup of coffee or tea. An ideal time for this would be after breakfast, although this time will not fit into every schedule. Learn, by experimenting, the foods and lifestyles that let you have bowel movements at a predictable time. Once you are having regular bowel movements, stick to the bowel program you developed. To quote a good nurse friend of mine, "Haste never makes waste." Find that special time.

If changing your diet and routine and using natural methods doesn't solve the problem of constipation, medications can be used. Your health care provider may suggest you try bulk formers, such as Metamucil, Perdiem, or FiberCon or other fiber pills. Stool softeners such as Colace or Surfak can help with hard stools. Your doctor may suggest a laxative but will likely prefer that you not become laxative dependent. Suppositories may be suggested in combination with other medications. Enemas may be necessary occasionally, but you need to avoid dependency on them, too.

Diarrhea, or loose stools, is much less common and is caused by diminished sphincter control or a hyperreflexic bowel. Bowel problems such as diarrhea are managed by diet, bowel training, and medications. In the event that loose stools become a problem, you would be referred to a gastroenterologist for consultation and treatment.

Vision

I woke up one morning a few weeks ago seeing two of everything. I couldn't even manage to dial the phone to our

ophthalmologist and had my husband do that. The ophthal-
mologist saw me right away and told me he was arranging
for me to see a neurologist at once. He thought I might be
having the first symptom of MS. Long story short—I have
what the neurologist terms "clinically isolated syndrome"
with an MRI [a magnetic resonance imaging scan] suspi-
cious for MS. I just finished my IV treatment.   CARLEY

Visual problems are often the first symptom people with MS have, the one that brings them to their doctor or ophthalmologist. You may be told that you have *optic neuritis*, which means that fibers of your optic nerve are inflamed. Pain and temporary vision loss are common symptoms of optic neuritis; you experience a loss of vision or your vision becomes imperfect. Up to fifty percent of patients with MS will develop an episode of optic neuritis. Your doctor will usually prescribe intravenous (IV) methylprednisolone, a steroid, for probably three to five days. Your treatment will be arranged at an infusion center or can be provided by a nursing agency in your home. A line will be introduced into a vein in your arm so that the steroid can drip through into the vein. If this is done in your home, you or a family member will learn how to infuse the drug. You will be taught what to look for that could indicate a problem and how to contact a nurse for help if needed.

Another potential visual problem is double vision. Diminished coordination and weakened eye muscles can cause double vision. When it comes on suddenly, it is usually treated with IV steroids, although your brain usually learns to compensate for double vision and images are eventually seen as normal.

Yet another visual problem could be *nystagmus*, or jerking eyes. This usually occurs when you look to the side; you may not even notice it. It usually is observed by your doctor when checking your eye movements during an evaluation of your vision. It is more of a nuisance than a major problem, although your doctor can prescribe a drug such as Klonopin (clonazepam) or Neurontin (gabapentin) if necessary.

What Nurses Know...

It is important for you to have regular eye examinations. MS may not be the cause of your eyesight problem; there are many other potential causes. However, the presence of demyelinating white matter lesions on a brain magnetic resonance imaging scan, accompanied by optic neuritis, is the strongest predictor for developing clinically definite MS.

Spasticity

The muscles in my thighs and calves are really stiff when I get up in the morning and sometimes off and on during the day. My MS nurse showed me how to do some stretching exercises right when I first get up and then at other times during the day when I feel stiff. They sure do make a difference.   LUKE

Spasticity, or stiffness, is a common problem in MS. Increased stiffness in the muscles caused by nerves that regulate muscle tone means that a great deal of energy is required to perform daily activities, and fatigue and incoordination result. Muscles are tight and resistant to stretch and may be painful. Spasticity is most often noted in the lower extremities, such as in the calf, thigh, buttocks, or groin. It affects walking or sleeping and worsens with infections, exacerbations, and constipation.

One of the first things to do if you notice spasticity is to develop a stretching regimen, which should include a series of exercises performed in certain sitting or lying positions that stretch specific muscles. After each muscle reaches its stretched position, hold it there for a minute to allow it to slowly relax. Begin at the ankle, stretching the calf muscles and then proceed upward to the muscles of the back of the thigh, the buttocks, and the groin.

What Nurses Know...

Exercising in a pool is beneficial because the water buoys you, and thus you expend less energy. The pool should be no warmer than 85°, because warm temperatures cause fatigue.

Mechanical aids, such as orthotics prescribed by a physical therapist or occupational therapist, may be used to control spasticity. These might include a "toe spreader" or "finger spreader" to relax tightness in toes or fingers or braces for the wrist, foot, or hand. A device for the foot might include an ankle-foot orthosis. These are usually custom made for each individual.

There are many medications used to manage spasticity. Unfortunately, most of them cause sleepiness and so are started at low doses and gradually increased until they provide relief. The more sedating medications are prescribed for bedtime. The medications most often used are Kemstro or Lioresal (baclofen) and Zanaflex (tizanidine), which are classified as antispasticity drugs. Other medications are used off label, such as Valium (diazepam), Klonopin (clonazepam), or Neurontin (gabapentin). For spasticity that is severely disabling and not responsive to oral drug therapy, intrathecal baclofen (i.e., delivered via a programmable pump surgically inserted into the abdominal wall) may provide relief. For spasticity that involves small groups of muscle an injection of Botox (OnabotulinumtoxinA) can provide relief. Spasticity can be managed in many ways, and medication is prescribed to fit the needs of the person experiencing it.

My husband complained that I kept him awake at night with my "jumping legs." When I mentioned this to my doctor, he prescribed some Zanaflex for me to take at night. My husband was no longer kept awake and I had a more restful night as well. MARILYN

Weakness

I really got upset because I felt increasing weakness in my arms and legs. I decided to put myself on a strenuous exercise program. I lifted weights and did a real workout on my stationary bike. I got weaker and weaker and more and more upset. I finally made an appointment with the physical therapist that my doctor had suggested for me to see and was told that I had been overexercising groups of muscles, causing them to become weaker. Now I am building strength with a proper exercise program and am feeling stronger JORDAN

In MS, weakness is caused by a problem in the transmission of electrical impulses to the muscle within the central nervous system (CNS). Weakness may come as an acute attack and may be treated with IV steroids, or it may progress slowly without any acute attacks. Exercises that involve repetitive movements or lifting weights to the point of fatigue increase weakness instead of increasing strength. It is very important that any exercises you do are appropriate for your situation. Your health care team needs to include a physical therapist who can teach you correct exercises to strengthen muscles, decrease weakness, and improve balance and coordination.

The physical therapist with whom you work needs to have a thorough understanding of MS and be able to suggest assistive devices that may help compensate for weak muscles and maintain your ability to walk. Physical therapy cannot cure the symptoms of MS, but it can enable you to counteract some of the changes brought about by MS. With all of the medications now available to treat MS symptoms, as well as those on the horizon, you probably won't need leg braces, a cane, or a wheelchair, but it is good to know that in the event that you might need them there are devices available that can help you maintain a quality of life that is acceptable to you. The right device, with your right attitude, can make all the difference.

Pain

Pain has historically not been attributed to MS, and yet we now know that people with MS do indeed experience pain. At least sixty-five to seventy percent of people with MS have experienced pain (Halper J, 2007). Pain makes no distinction regarding how long you have had MS, your age at onset, or your gender. What we all must remember is that pain is whatever you say it is and exists whenever you say it does. MS itself may cause pain, or the pain may be secondary to your having MS, or it may result from some of the treatments you are using for MS. It may be acute, sudden, or intense, relating to demyelination, such as pain in trigeminal neuralgia (a severe, stabbing facial pain), optic neuritis, or migraine or tension headaches, or it may be secondary pain, related to an exacerbation or weakness in or improper use of compensatory muscles. It could be associated with a UTI or stress on bones as a result of weakness, deconditioning or improper use of compensatory muscles. It can be chronic musculoskeletal pain related to your disease. It can be pain caused by spasticity, or what is called *dyesthetic pain*, meaning pain that feels like burning or prickling, a "pins and needles" sensation, or it can comprise nagging, dull, or band-like sensations in legs, feet, arms or trunk. You may have pain related to a relapse. You may experience pain that is not related to your MS. As I mentioned earlier, and will repeat over and over in this book, MS does not exempt one from other illnesses, such as arthritis, dental problems, back problems, cancer, or accidents. Psychological symptoms correlating with poor mood and depression can result in emotional pain. The first step in dealing with pain is to determine its cause.

Trigeminal neuralgia is a severe, stabbing facial pain that is occasionally seen in individuals with MS. Anticonvulsants, which are drugs used for epilepsy, are used for this condition. Examples might be Tegretol (carbamazepine), Keppra (levetiracetam),

Trileptal (oxcarbazepine), Gabitril (tiagabine), or Neurontin. If these medications don't control the pain, a surgical procedure may be performed.

L'Hermitte's sign is the term used for an unusual electrical sensation that it felt down the spine and into the legs when the neck is moved. This is a momentary sensation and is not significant in terms of predicting the course of MS, although it is a bothersome symptom when it occurs. Another type of pain is what we call the MS "hug," or a girdle-band sensation in which you feel like you have a band around your middle.

Probably the most common type of pain experienced in MS is a burning-type pain that occurs most often in the arms and legs but may also occur on the trunk. Antiepileptic medications such as those used for trigeminal neuralgia (e.g., Tegretol, Neurontin, Trileptal, Keppra) may be prescribed. Antidepressants are used off label for this pain because they alter the interpretation of the message of pain. Do not assume if you are prescribed one that it is because your practitioner thinks your pain is "all in your head." The best-known antidepressants used for burning pain are Elavil, Pamelor, and Tofranil (imipramine). Cymbalta (Duloxetine) is used for neuropathic pain with MS because it treats both depression and pain.

Spasticity causes pain. Treatments for spasticity were discussed earlier in this chapter. Poor walking patterns caused by other MS symptoms can result in pain and may be treated with an exercise program or an assistive device. Topical medications such as lidocaine or capsaicin, as well as heat and cold compresses, may be helpful.

Standard pain medications, such as nonsteroidal anti-inflammatory drugs (NSAIDs), may be helpful in treating pain. In general, health care practitioners try to not use narcotic medications for MS. Not only are they not usually effective but also, and more important, they are addictive or habit forming and result in increasing doses. Cannabis (marijuana) has been reported by some individuals to benefit MS symptoms, but its effects have been short lived, and it has a potential for abuse and tolerance. Studies are underway to test cannabis for various MS symptoms, but the jury is still out. In 2009, the National Multiple Sclerosis Society released recommendations regarding marijuana as a treatment for MS. Their official statement said, in part: "Although it is clear that cannabinoids have a potential for both management of MS symptoms such as pain and spasticity, as well as for neuroprotection," it cannot yet be recommended because "studies to date do not demonstrate a clear benefit compared to existing symptomatic therapies and... issues of side effects, systemic effects and long-term effects are not yet clear." We are all waiting for more evidence.

In using pain medications health care professionals usually start at a low dose and gradually work up to a dose that is effective. If partial relief occurs with one drug, a combination of two or more different classes of drugs can often yield better results. In general, when one is pain free or three months on a treatment regimen, your doctor will consider slowly tapering you off the medication.

What Nurses Know ...

Pain causes associated symptoms and must be treated. Some of these symptoms include

- *Insomnia*
- *Anxiety*
- *Depression*
- *Weight loss or gain*
- *Disturbed relationships with family members and friends*

Sexual Problems

As a disease that affects your CNS, MS lesions and their location certainly can be the cause of sexual symptoms. Males can experience problems with erections and ejaculation. Drugs such as Viagra (sildenafil) and Cialis (tadalafil) are very helpful for men with erectile problems. If these drugs don't work, your urologist may prescribe Caverject (alprostadil urogenital), which can be injected into the penis thirty minutes before intercourse, or Muse (alprostadil injectable and transurethral), which is administered into the opening of the penis. Women can experience a lack of feeling in their genital area and a lack of vaginal lubrication and diminished orgasmic response. Lubricants such as Replens or Astroglide (never use Vaseline) and vibrators are helpful. Sexual difficulties are very serious problems because they affect relationships and marriages and the way people feel about their sexuality. I discuss sexuality further in Chapter 7 in my discussion of MS and the family and relationships.

Cognition

I just can't remember the way I used to. I make lists and then forget where I left my list. I don't get to the places I need to be. I forgot all about my son's soccer tournament, and I was in charge of drinks and snacks for that. We don't entertain anymore because I simply can't get an entire meal together. I try to blame my problem on the fact that I am getting older, but I am only 32. My husband is at his wits' end not knowing how to help me and suggested that I talk with the neurologist about this problem. My neurologist was able to blame MS for this problem, and sent me for what he termed neuropsychological testing. *The neuropsychologist who worked with me was wonderful and gave John and me suggestions that help. She says I have trouble multitasking, and now we break everything down so that I just have to follow through on one thing at a time. I also have a basket in the kitchen for my lists. It is red and I can't miss it.   PATSY*

I remember attending a meeting with a group of neurologists some twenty years ago and hearing one neurologist say "Well, at least I tell my MS patients that MS doesn't affect their cognition." I almost fell out of my seat! Cognition comprises thinking skills, understanding language and expression of thoughts and ideas, concentrating, multitasking, learning and remembering new information, and solving problems. The people I work with who have MS complain of problems with all of these things. They are actually relieved to learn that they can blame these problems on their MS. Cognitive impairment among individuals with MS are wide ranging but and it has been estimated that seventy percent of people with MS complain of some cognitive problems at some time during the course of their disease (Wilken JA, Sullivan C, Mitchell W, et al. 2008). They can come and go like other MS symptoms. Cognitive problems are not related to physical disability and may occur early in the disease. They have even been known as the problem that brings some people to their doctors to eventually be diagnosed with MS.

Problems with cognition can affect the way you are able to manage your household or take care of your family. Cognitive problems certainly affect relationships and social interactions and whether or not you are able to perform in your job. Being able to function well cognitively is one of the things we value most and something that none of us wants to lose. It is important to know that the cognitive problems experienced by people who live with MS differ from those experienced by people who have Alzheimer's disease. MS exerts selective effects on cognitive function and, unlike in Alzheimer's, MS cognitive impairment appears to be relatively stable over time.

What Nurses Know...

I once ran across what one anonymous person with MS wrote about her cognitive problem. Many of my patients and their family members are able to relate:I decided to wash my car. As I start toward the garage, I notice that there is mail on the hall table. I decide to go through the mail before I wash the car. I lay my car keys down on the table, put the junk mail in the trash can under the table, and notice that the trash can is full. So, I decide to put the bills back on the table and take out the trash first, but then I think, since I am going to be near the mailbox when I take out the trash anyway, I may as well pay the bills first. I take my checkbook off the table and see that there is only one check left. My extra checks are in my desk in the study, so I go to my desk where I find a can of Coke that I had been drinking. I am going to look for my checks, but first I need to push the Coke aside so that I don't accidentally knock it over. I see that the Coke is getting warm and decide I should put it in the refrigerator to keep it cold. As I head toward the kitchen with the Coke, a vase of flowers on the counter catches my eye—they need to be watered. I set the Coke down on the counter and discover my reading glasses that I've been searching for all morning. I decide I better put them back on my desk, but first I'm going to water the flowers. I set the glasses back down on the counter, fill a container with water, and suddenly I spot the TV remote. Someone left it on the kitchen table. I realize that tonight when we go to watch TV, we will be looking for the remote, but nobody will remember that it's on the kitchen table, so I decide to put it back in the den where it belongs, but first I'll water the flowers. I splash some water on the flowers, but most of it spills on the floor.

So, I set the remote back down on the table, get some towels and wipe up the spill. Then I head down the hall trying to remember what I was planning to do.

At the end of the day, the car isn't washed, the bills aren't paid, there is a warm can of Coke sitting on the counter, the flowers aren't watered, there is still only one check in my checkbook, I can't find the remote, I can't find my glasses, and I don't remember what I did with the car keys. Then when I try to figure out why nothing got done today, I am really baffled because I know I was busy all day long and I'm really tired!

What are some of the things that make you feel that you may be experiencing problems with cognition? Symptoms may include one or more of the following:

- Memory dysfunction
- Difficulty following directions
- Difficulty making decisions
- Being slow to understand what you hear
- Poor verbal fluency
- Poor performance at work
- Difficulty starting or finishing a project, following a recipe, or balancing your checkbook

Certainly MS lesions in your brain may be the cause of your cognitive symptoms, but there are conditions not related to MS that may cause symptoms such as these. Physical fatigue can bring about mental fatigue, which may slow your speed in processing information, in accuracy, and in reaction time. Depression certainly affects your memory. Stress can play a big part in cognition. Keep in mind that some of the medications you take for other problems may dull your cognitive function. You may not realize that you are having problems, but your family members may note that things have changed.

> *I had a terrible time just trying to get a meal prepared and doing normal tasks around the house. This caused real frustration for my husband and for me. When I had neuro-psychological testing this came out as a real problem. My husband and I were shown by the neuropsychologist how tasks could be broken down into parts and I could follow directions to do one thing at a time. I could do things, and this made a real difference in our family life.* CAROLYN

When you or your family notes that you are showing some signs that might indicate cognitive dysfunction, you need to bring this up to your health care provider., who can refer you to a neuropsychologist for cognitive testing. You will be evaluated to determine the cause of your problems. Fortunately, a good neuropsychologist will make you aware of your strengths as well as any weaknesses and will arrange for some therapy to help you know how to live with and make up for things that are problematic. You may work with a neuropsychologist, a speech-language pathologist, or an occupational therapist.

Once again, MS is a disease of the CNS, which governs all the nerve impulses in your body. I have discussed the most common symptoms people with MS might have, but there are certainly other symptoms that can be caused by the demyelination that characterizes this disease. Symptoms can be intermittent or continual, and some may worsen. The therapies health care providers use need to be geared to what you are experiencing and flexible enough to change when the symptom does. Please do not hesitate to share with your MS nurse or neurologist anything that you think may be a symptom. They can decide with you whether you need treatment and what that treatment should be.

References

Halper J. (2007). Advanced Concepts in Multiple Sclerosis Nursing Care, Second Editon, New York, Demos Medical Publishing.

Kalb RC. (2008). Multiple Sclerosis: The Questions You Have, The Answers You Need. Fourth Edition, New York, Demos Medical Publishing.

Oken BS, Kishiyama MA, Zajdel D. et al. Randomized controlled trial of yoga and exercise in multiple sclerosis. *Neurology*, Arch Intern Med. 2010;170(4):321-331.

Patten SB. (2009) *Antidepressant Treatment for Major Depression in Multilple Sclerosis.* International Journal of MS Care, 11:4, 174.

Rogers RG. (2008). Urinary Stress Incontinence in Women. N Engl J Med, 358:1029-1036.

Wilken JA, Sullivan C, Mitchell W, et al. (2008). *Treatment of Multiple Sclerosis-Related Cognitive Problems With Adjunctive Modafinil.* International Journal of MS Care, 10:1.

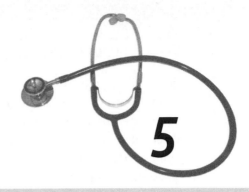

Treating an Exacerbation or Relapse

I woke up this morning and just couldn't get out of bed. I had been up most of the night running to the bathroom, and now I couldn't get out of bed to make it there in time. When I called my multiple sclerosis nurse and talked with her about my symptoms, she insisted that I get a urine culture. I had a urinary tract infection, and when that was treated, all of my weakness went away. MARLA

All of a sudden on my way home from work, the day before yesterday, my vision started to blur. It was no better yesterday, so I stayed home from work and rested. Today it is still blurred. My doctor had me come into the office, checked my vision, and sent me to the infusion center for steroids. KAREN

Multiple sclerosis (MS) relapses are one of the most frustrating things about this disease for people living with MS, their doctors, and their loved ones to deal with and understand. The terms *exacerbation* or *relapse* mean the same thing and are used interchangeably. An exacerbation or relapse, sometimes referred to as a *flare*, must include one or more neurological symptoms, must last more than twenty-four hours, and must not be secondary to an infection or fever. True relapses usually last several weeks, although they can be as short as a couple of days or as long as several months. When you call your health care provider to report symptoms that you feel might be a relapse, you will be asked to describe your symptoms and indicate how long you have been experiencing them. Then you will be asked if you are experiencing a cough or cold, or any pain on urination or sudden change in urinary frequency. Infections can cause a "pseudo relapse" that is not related to new disease activity but can aggravate the neurologic effects of preexisting plaques. When these infections are treated, the MS symptoms return to their previous level. It is important to determine the cause of your symptoms. If the symptoms you are reporting sound like they may be a relapse, your doctor will probably want to examine you and will arrange to have you come in for an appointment.

What could an exacerbation look like? Symptoms include any of the following:

- Numbness or weakness
- Constant fatigue
- Loss of muscle function
- Problems with memory and attention
- Urinary issues
- Tremors or muscle spasms
- Problems with walking or balance
- Difficulty speaking
- Changes in vision
- Facial pain

A symptom can be a flare up of an old symptom or a completely new symptom.

MS relapses are usually treated with high-dose steroids such as intravenous (IV) methylprednisolone (brand name Solu-Medrol), oral prednisone, Decadron (dexamethasone) or Acthar Gel (corticotropin). These are given to decrease inflammation in the area of demyelination so that the impulses going to the brain return to normal and your symptoms subside. Again, they are not a cure for MS, but they may put an end to your relapse.

If you and your physician decide on a treatment with methylprednisolone, you will receive your treatment at an infusion center or in your home by making arrangements with a home health care agency. If a home health care agency provides your treatment in your home, a nurse will bring the equipment needed for your infusions, put a line in your arm, and infuse your first treatment. The nurse will work with you or a family member to learn to give the remainder of your infusions once a day for the three to five days ordered by your doctor. If your treatment takes place at an infusion center, you will go there for the three to five days that your doctor has ordered treatment. Your IV treatment may or may not be followed by an oral steroid treatment with prednisone or Decadron given in decreasing doses for several days. Your doctor may decide to give you only oral steroids for several days. If you are someone who has very poor venous access and it is very difficult for a nurse to introduce an IV, you may be prescribed Acthar Gel, a steroid that can be given by subcutaneous or intramuscular injection. Because Acthar Gel is very expensive, it is reserved for special situations, for example, if you have had an allergic reaction to methylprednisolone, or have had difficulty tolerating methylprednisolone, or you have veins that are difficult to access if Solumedrol has not been effective for you, or if you are unable to get to an infusion center and a home health care agency is not available.

I have been diagnosed with MS. My husband is in the military, and we move around so often that I don't have one neurologist who can help manage my MS. About a year ago I had what I thought must be a flare of my MS. My legs were so weak that I could barely walk at all. This was the first time I had experienced anything since I was diagnosed two years earlier. I found a neurologist who could see me and he felt this was an exacerbation that needed to be treated with steroids. He arranged for me to have Solu-Medrol in my home since I did not live near an infusion center. A nurse from a home health agency came to the house, put a line in my arm and started my first infusion. After half an hour I was covered with a red rash. The nurse called my doctor, who said to stop the infusion and that he would order Decadron, which I could take orally once the rash had disappeared. I started the Decadron, and after my second dose, the rash was back. My doctor said that he felt I was a candidate for a trial with Acthar Gel. My insurance approved this treatment, and a nurse came out to my home to show my husband and me how to give me injections of the drug. That part was no problem since I already take injections of Rebif three days a week. After five days of Acthar, I was walking well again, and best of all I did not have a rash. My doctor gave me a letter stating that I had had an allergic reaction to both IV Solu-Medrol and Decadron and that for future exacerbations I should be prescribed Acthar Gel. That gives me a sense of control as we move about the country. FLORRIE

Steroids can make your symptoms subside so that you function as you did before your relapse, or at least at a level acceptable to you. However, as with most medications, they have side effects. Steroids may make you have high or low mood changes.

What Nurses Know...

Treatment with steroids can shorten relapses, but their side effects don't make them anyone's favorite medication.

They can make you feel so strong that you feel as though you could "jump over buildings with a single bound" or can make you want to eat everything in sight. Often you are so invigorated that you can't sleep at night. I've had women who say that they are up cleaning their house at night and have run out of things to do. I have offered them the opportunity to clean my house, but as yet no one has taken me up on that offer!

My wife is impossible when she has a relapse and is put on steroids. I have to remind myself and the rest of the family that she is not herself and will return to the woman and mom that we all love and respect once these infusions are over. It has made me realize that I need to help her with her injections of Copaxone to keep her from forgetting to do them so as to try to reduce the times she needs to be on steroids. ALLEN

It is important that you get your rest, so if you have an overly energetic reaction to a steroid you will need something prescribed to help you sleep at night. Your doctor may prescribe a drug such as Ambien (zolpidem) or Lunesta (eszopiclone) to help you sleep. Steroids also may cause stomach discomfort, and you may be told to take something like Maalox or Zantac to prevent this. Steroids make some people feel weak and tired and nauseated and unable to eat much at all. Health care professionals are not able to predict which reaction you will have.

I just love being on steroids. They make me feel so "up." I have energy to do everything. I try to let my doctor know of anything that could possibly be caused by my MS and hope that he will prescribe some steroids for me. I know that long term they may cause problems, but I want to live for now, and they make me feel so good. CLAUDIA

Please don't give me steroids again. Taking them is worse than suffering with a bad symptom. They make me feel nauseated, and I don't even want to get out of bed. I am just not able to function as the mom of the family. Even the kids remind me to take my shot every other day. They don't want me to have to take steroids ever again. LORNA

Because your kidneys are getting rid of potassium, it is recommended that you eat foods high in potassium, such as orange juice, tomatoes, green leafy vegetables, or cantaloupe. If you get really hungry while on steroids and overeat, you will probably gain weight and not be happy with yourself.

I was doing really well after my diagnosis, with no problems at all, and then all of a sudden I was numb from my waist down. I was so upset and scared. My doctor ordered IV steroids with a home health care agency. I forgot all about how my doctor warned me to cut out the salt in my diet. I guess I just couldn't remember all he said because I was so worried about my symptoms. When I am worried, I eat. I ate everything I could find, lots of chips and junk. I put on way too many pounds, and they took weeks to shed. I know now that if I have to take steroids again, I will watch my diet for salt and for eating too much because I don't what that weight gain. JANET

What Nurses Know...

Watch that salt! When your system is flooded with high-dose steroids, your adrenal glands, which make corticosteroids in your body, stop making them and send a message to your kidneys to save sodium and get rid of potassium. The sodium combines with water and can cause you to retain water, so you may note some bloating. Thus, your health care professional likely will tell you not to eat foods high in sodium while you are on steroids.

Long-term use of steroids can cause long-range problems like osteoporosis, diabetes, bone loss, hypertension, cataracts, and ulcers. For both sexes, increased aggressiveness, otherwise known as "roid rage," commonly accompanies the use of steroids. It is recommended that adults with MS get a dexa scan to measure baseline bone density early after their MS diagnosis, have routine follow-up scans over time, and eat a diet rich in calcium.

Prevention

As we discussed earlier, some MS drugs can alter the course of the disease by slowing its progression. Again, all of these drugs are different from one another to some degree, and you will need to work with your health care provider to pick the one that is right for you. Before these treatments existed people relied on corticosteroids to shorten relapses, medications for specific symptoms, and physical and occupational therapy to adjust to and slow disability. These treatments are still used, but health care professionals believe that the disease-modifying drugs do actually modify the course of MS. When you are on immunotherapy, you likely will have fewer, and milder, relapses and less disability overall. So the first and most important thing that you can do to prevent relapses is to begin using, and adhere to, one of the disease-modifying therapies.

However, in all honesty, and as I mentioned earlier, the course MS will take is not something one can predict. Should the number or rate of relapses increase, you and your neurologist can decide to use some treatments that have not been approved for MS but that have been known to help some people, such as IV immunoglobin or Cytoxan (cyclophosphamide) infusions, or drugs such as Imuran (azathioprine), methotrexate (e.g., Rheumatrex), or CellCept (mycophenolate). Your neurologist also may suggest a change to another immunotherapy. What health care professionals call *pulse steroids*—steroids given one or two days monthly or every other month to prevent relapses—is another treatment that might be used. Whatever option you choose, there will be a health care team ready to make suggestions to help you decide on treatments and to live in a way that it acceptable to you.

Certainly when you have a relapse you can feel like it is the end of the world. You want your disease to be under control, and you don't want to be disabled. You believe that if you have frequent relapses, you are going to become disabled. I cannot guarantee that you are wrong, but health care providers' ultimate goal is to reduce those relapses and give you time to live the life you want. They will encourage you to be adherent to your immunotherapy regimen and be a member of the "never miss a dose club." You will have some symptoms and relapses, reminders of MS, but your doctor will work with you to make those few and far between, sometimes adding other medications if necessary or switching to a different therapy. Your MS team will work with you and with your family to give you the care that you need.

> *I work with a gal who has MS. We go to the same MS center for our care and love to compare notes. My friend started an immunotherapy as soon as she had some symptoms and hasn't even had a flare that needed treatment. For me it has been a different story. I have tried all of the immunotherapies out there and not been able to tolerate any of them. I couldn't stand the flu like symptoms and hated to have red spots on my body. I would just stop the drug I was taking and suffer from symptoms that usually needed treatment with steroids. Then I would go for another therapy which I wouldn't like either. I think my doctor is about ready to give up on me. We are talking about Tysabri or Gilenya and I am reading up. I really am grateful that the staff at my MS center continues to work with someone as difficult as I must be. MARY ELLEN*

Multiple sclerosis is difficult to live with and difficult to treat. There is no cure and we want to work with you to have the life you want. We are grateful for the therapies that certainly have made a difference and have come to us during the past sixteen years and we look forward to more in the near future. All have some side effects that must be considered. All take some effort on your part to tolerate. Until we have a cure there will be relapses and there will be treatment with steroids.

Multiple Sclerosis Exacerbations and Your Feelings

It is thought that an association exists between stress and MS, but stress in and of itself probably does not precipitate an MS exacerbation. Everyone wants to live their lives to the fullest, including people who have multiple sclerosis. But it's hard to do that when you are thinking about what may happen or what may not happen next. Early in your MS diagnosis you may live in fear of exacerbations. One of the things that make MS a unique condition is the progressive nature of it. It's not a static, stable condition, and it varies so much from person to person. So there is no road map as to what you should expect with your MS. This adds a lot more fear and worry for people living with MS. Our minds are really incredibly powerful tools, and controlling thoughts can help then to control our emotions. What you think has a direct bearing on how you feel. So fight to stay positive.

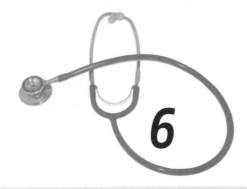

6

Multiple Sclerosis and Complementary and Alternative Medicine

My friends keep telling me about things they have heard help multiple sclerosis (MS) and telling me to try them. The clerks at the health food store have lots more suggestions. One of my friends brought me some midnight primrose oil that a friend told her was really helpful for people with MS. Since there is no cure, should I look into some of these things?   MABEL

All the medications out for MS are really expensive, and they aren't cures. I have heard about lots of "natural" things that are lots cheaper, and I think I am just going to try them. I figure that I have nothing to lose and maybe something to gain.   NOAH

Alternative therapies are nonmedical interventions that are used instead of conventional medical therapy. They are not usually provided by your doctor or available in hospitals. *Complementary therapies* are used in conjunction with conventional therapies.

Although the various therapies are all different, the major complementary and alternative medicine (CAM) therapies have some common characteristics that include a focus on individualizing treatments, treating the whole person, promoting self-care and self-healing, and sometimes an involvement of the spiritual nature of us as people. Conventional medicine does not have all of the answers, and people want to do all that they can to promote their own health and be proactive patients.

CAM therapies allow people living with multiple sclerosis (MS) to promote better overall health for themselves, to be proactive. MS is chronic and usually progressive and, as I have stated before, there is no medical cure yet available for it, although we are ever hopeful. In interviewing people who would come to our MS center wanting to be included in investigational studies my colleagues and I were conducting, I would ask what medications they were taking and would get a list of medications commonly used to treat MS symptoms. When I asked the person being interviewed about medications he or she was taking that were obtained over the counter, without a prescription, I would get another list, often longer than the first.

In a Rocky Mountain MS Center survey alternative therapies are used by at least four out of every ten adults in the general population, and billions of dollars are spent on alternative treatments each year (Bowling AC, 2007). Fortunately, CAM is

What Nurses Know...

It is of extreme importance to disclose to your medical provider everything you are taking, including all vitamins, herbs, and holistic medicines. There can be bad interactions between these and your prescribed drugs. Just because they are "natural" does not mean they are always harmless.

usually used in conjunction with conventional medicine, with only a few people using it in a truly alternative manner. This is especially true when CAM includes dietary supplements, special diets, acupuncture, meditation, chiropractic medicine, massage, and yoga.

In considering a CAM therapy one needs to take time to gather information on the therapy under consideration. Certainly you can seek out books on this topic. Allen Bowling, MD, PhD, from the Rocky Mountain MS Center in Englewood, Colorado, has written an outstanding resource on the subject, *Complementary and Alternative Medicine and Multiple Sclerosis.* None of the various CAM therapies have been approved by the Food and Drug Administration; however, you naturally will want to know that a therapy is safe and that there is some evidence that it might be helpful in regard to the purpose for which you want to use it. When you decide to use a CAM therapy, talk with your health care team and see that your doctor has that product on your list of medications, because there could be possible interactions with conventional therapies. "Natural" does not mean safe. Some natural therapies are safe and beneficial, and some are toxic. "Over the counter" does not mean safe, either. Anything you take may have side effects. It is important that you learn as much as

What Nurses Know...

The following are some guidelines to consider when choosing a CAM therapy:
- *Is there any evidence that it is harmful?*
- *Is there any evidence that it is helpful?*
- *Is it too expensive for my budget?*
- *Is it too difficult to access?*
- *Does it sound too good to be true?*

possible about any alternative or complementary medications you consider taking. You need to know more than the fact that the clerk at the health food store, who is working his or her way through high school, suggests this or that supplement for you.

Lots of herbs have been shown to activate the immune system and thus worsen MS symptoms. Other herbs can irritate the urinary tract and worsen the symptoms of urinary tract infections. Some herbs may interact with steroids, antidepressant medications, or interferons, so they need to be used with caution. Herbs are biologically based, as are vitamins, nutritional supplements, and bee sting therapy. Bee sting therapy was a popular CAM treatment for MS several years ago. People claimed that with regular bee stings (bee venom) they could manage some of the symptoms of MS.

Alternative medical systems include acupuncture and homeopathy. Mind and body medicine, which also comprises alternative therapies, includes relaxation methods, tai chi, yoga, spirituality, hypnotherapy, and laughter. Manipulative and body-based systems include chiropractic; massage; reflexology; and energy therapies, including therapeutic touch and magnet therapy.

Chiropractic is widely used in MS and has been associated with reported benefits in pain relief and well-being. A survey on the former web site, www.ms-cam.org yielded responses indicating benefits in pain, anxiety, depression, muscle stiffness, and fatigue. Chiropractic care can help to alleviate musculoskeletal symptoms associated with MS, such as spasticity, joint contractures, or other secondary problems caused by the disease. People with MS experience a varying degree of relief, albeit temporary, from their musculoskeletal symptoms by seeing a chiropractor. This is a quality of life issue: If something can provide you with some form of relief, even if it is for your secondary symptoms, then it can be of value.

A friend of mine suggested that I add kava kava to my medication regimen. I tend to be anxious about so many things, especially anything connected with my MS. I didn't notice that I became less anxious once I started taking it, but I felt sedated all the time and could hardly stay awake. I mentioned that I was taking kava kava to my doctor who told me that it has a sedating effect when taken with medications such as baclofen and Zanaflex, which I take for spasticity. My doctor also pointed out that it could cause liver toxicity and that I would need regular labs to check for this if I decided to continue taking the drug. I stopped taking kava kava and shall be careful before I try something else. MALCOLM

Another survey on the former web site www.ms-cam.org that addressed cannabis (which continues to be illegal in most of the United States) stated that patients reported a benefit of pain and spasticity but worsening symptoms in speech, anxiety, thinking problems, balance, and fatigue.

I've heard several people talk about how using low-dose naltrexone can be beneficial to people with MS. I decided to ask my doctor about giving me a prescription. My doctor pointed out that there are no clinical trials that have evaluated naltrexone for safety and effectiveness. He advised that further studies are needed since we believe in evidence-based medication. I decided I wouldn't take it. AL

Naltrexone is a drug that has attracted a lot of buzz in the MS community. The problem is that no formal studies have been conducted that prove or disprove that it works. We continue to lack the kind of evidence that physicians need to prescribe it for MS. Naltrexone is an opioid receptor antagonist that is used primarily in the management of alcohol dependence and opioid dependence. It is marketed in generic form as its hydrochloride salt, called *naltrexone hydrochloride*, and sold under the trade names ReVia and Depade. Low-dose naltrexone, a form in which the drug is used in doses approximately

one-tenth of those used for drug/alcohol rehabilitation purposes, is being used by some health care professionals as an
off-label experimental treatment for various disorders, including not only MS but also HIV/AIDS, Parkinson's disease, cancer, fibromyalgia, and others. Again, there are no long-term
studies to judge the efficacy or the long-term effects of this
drug on people with MS.

> *I've heard that drinking cranberry juice will keep me from
> having urinary tract infections, which are so common in
> MS. My doctor says that cranberry juice shouldn't be used
> to treat urinary tract infections but may be reasonable in
> preventing infections. Drinking high doses could cause kid-
> ney stones. I like cranberry juice, so I intend to keep drink-
> ing it in moderation.*   MEGHAN

There has been much talk about the prevalence of vitamin D
deficiency in the U.S. population and evidence of low levels of
vitamin D in people with MS. One study indicated that levels of
vitamin D may be lower in people with MS during relapses. In
an examination of magnetic resonance imaging scan activity,
researchers noted that MS may vary with the seasons, with more
lesions in the winter and fewer in the summer, when there is
more sun (and thus more vitamin D exposure). One study found
that women who took vitamin D supplements were less likely to
develop MS (www.nmss.org).

What Nurses Know...

*Drink cranberry juice or use cranberry tablets to help main-
tain urinary tract health, but NOT if you have a personal or
family history of kidney stones.*

What Nurses Know...

Even if there were not large bodies of research relating MS to vitamin D deficiency, there is plenty of evidence pointing to a vitamin D deficiency in the population as a whole. Sun exposure to the skin is the cheapest and most efficient way of getting adequate amounts of vitamin D. If you have MS and cannot tolerate the sun, talk to your doctor about vitamin D supplements.

Vitamin D use in people with MS is currently being studied, and it is recommended that patients be tested for vitamin D levels and take vitamin D supplements if their levels are low. Adequate levels of vitamin D are important because, along with calcium, they are important in maintaining bone density, which can be affected by steroid use. Low levels of vitamin D are noted these days in people with other diseases and in the general population, perhaps because we are learning to spend less time in the sun as a way to prevent skin cancer. Certainly people with MS reduce their exposure to the sun because they are so affected by heat.

Diet

Eating a balanced diet when you have MS is important, and diet should be considered in any discussion of nonmedical treatments and MS. One of the first things that patients who are newly diagnosed with MS usually want to know is if there is a specific diet for MS. So often we are told that we can control a disease with the proper diet. Health care professionals would like to be able to do that for MS. Unfortunately, there is no conclusive scientific evidence to show that any one nutritional therapy affects the course of MS. We know that sensible eating habits have a dramatic beneficial impact on general health and that maintaining a healthy body weight, along with good nutrition, is crucial. Steroid use and other medications used in MS can foster weight gain, as can a sedentary lifestyle caused by disability. It is important to plan weight control through nutrition and exercise.

The Swank Diet was developed by Dr. Ray Swank during the 1940s for people with MS. The diet was low in saturated fats, excluded high-fat dairy products, and called for frequent fish meals. There were few risks with this diet, but it was very hard to follow, and no studies have been conducted to prove that it made a difference in MS. There have been modifications of this diet, and some people with MS follow these modified diets. Diets are now getting a lot of attention in the MS community. As with most diets, there is not a lot of evidence to support their efficacy, but if a diet is not extreme there usually is no harm in trying it. Check with your doctor first about any diet you want to try, and do your research!

It is essential for people who have MS to have a healthy diet that includes at least three meals each day, starting with breakfast, and no skipped meals. Your diet should include a wide variety of foods based on the Dietary Guidelines for Americans released by the U.S. Department of Health and Human Services in 2005 (see http://www.mypyramid.gov/guidelines/index.html). Updated 2010 guidelines are in development but, as of this writing, have not yet been released.

The guidelines include the following recommendations:

- Make selections from the five basic food groups of the pyramid that emphasize food high in complex carbohydrate—three or more ounces of whole grains and a variety of fruits and vegetables.
- Eat fiber-rich foods
- Make sure that less than ten percent of the calories you eat are from saturated fats.
- Eat low-fat dairy foods, because dairy products are high in fat.

- Bake, broil, and boil your food instead of frying it, and eat lean cuts of meat. Limit meat to three or four ounces per day, and include skinless poultry and ocean fish (e.g., tuna, swordfish).
- Reduce simple sugar intake. Simple sugars are the refined sugars found in table sugars and in sweets like cookies, cakes and candy.
- Drink six to eight glasses of water each day.
- Limit your sodium intake, using seasonings to replace salt in foods.
- Maintain a total fat intake of between twenty and thirty-five percent of the calories you consume.
- Learn to read food labels.
- Emphasize portion size.

If you stick to these guidelines you will give yourself the benefit of a sound diet and contribute to your total health.

I am one of these guys trying to make my way up the career ladder. Before being diagnosed with MS at age 25 I skipped breakfast, often skipped lunch or got something fast at the deli, and then almost always stopped for fast food on my way home at night. Along with being told that I have MS I was instructed that I needed to have three square meals each day, low in fat and salt and starting with breakfast. I made the big change, and I have to say that I feel much better, and it really isn't hard to do. I even find time three times a week to visit the gym. When my mom found out about how I am eating she said that a diagnosis of MS wasn't all bad. JERRY

I have already discussed the importance of exercise when you have MS. You need to develop an exercise program that is the correct one for you and follow it. A physical therapist or fitness coach who is trained in MS may help you. Proper exercise increases fitness and reduces fatigue. You need to use aerobic and strengthening exercise for the proper length of time with the proper frequency and intensity. You really can't determine all of this by yourself. If you exercise too strenuously, fatigue and weakness will increase, so you need a program that is tailored to your individual needs.

Yoga can be adapted for people with MS who have disability. It is an outstanding kind of activity because it exercises the mind, body, and spirit using breathing, meditation, and posture. It provides positive emotional benefits as well as physical benefits, such as increased strength and improved muscle stretch and balance. I often bring yoga instructors who are or want to become knowledgeable about MS to MS support group meetings, and they design and arrange for group yoga sessions. Find instructors in your area and join a yoga class.

Tai chi is a form of Chinese martial arts that comprises exercise that can improve balance and coordination and increase strength as well as promote emotional balance. It is widely practiced by people with MS and can be adapted for people with disabilities. Tai chi programs are slow and controlled, with periodic changes in positions. It is relaxing and requires mental discipline and controlled breathing. This is another form of exercise for you to look into.

Until there is a cure for MS, and until all symptoms of MS have been resolved, people with MS will use every means they

What Nurses Know...

According to researchers at Oregon Health & Science University, yoga did not influence cognitive function or mood in their study, but it did lessen fatigue and increase energy level (Haupt 2007).

What Nurses Know...

According to the National MS Society, "Recent clinical studies have confirmed that tai chi produces measurable benefits in improving balance, lowering blood pressure and improving cardiovascular health. None of these studies involved people with MS, however." Researchers at the University of Brighton conducted a primary study on tai chi with favorable enough results that they are conducting a secondary one. The pilot study was funded by the MS Research Trust (www.msrc.co.uk).

can to alleviate their symptoms. Health care teams will suggest CAM therapies such as yoga and physical therapy exercise, as well as good basic nutrition, with supplements when needed. Be cautioned, however, that you cannot substitute CAM therapies for conventional therapies. Look for evidence that any CAM therapy you are considering is not harmful. Look for evidence that it could be helpful. Don't spend money on alternative therapies that would be more wisely spent on evidence-based treatment. When someone tells you something like goat serum from goats inoculated with vaccines generate neutralizing antibodies that are "potentially useful" in MS, toss the information aside until there is published research evidence to support the claim. (This advice comes from Patricia Kennedy, RN, CNP, MSCN, from Can Do MS.) All of your friends have their eyes out for helpful information that they will share with you. Do your research, choose wisely, and share anything you decide to do with your medical team.

References

Bowling, A. C. (2007). Complementary and Alternative Medicine and Multiple Sclerosis, Second Edition, New York, Demos Medical Publishing, 8-10.

Haupt J. (2007). Mindful of Pain. *Neurology Now.* November/ December 3:6, 20-27.

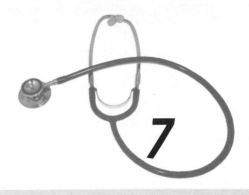

Multiple Sclerosis and Your Family, Your Friends, and Your Workplace

I have multiple sclerosis (MS) and I know I am going to have to share that fact with my family and perhaps some of my friends—or maybe I don't want friends to know. Do I have to let my superiors at my workplace know that I have MS?   RUSS

Why does multiple sclerosis (MS) have such an impact on others? The following are some reasons:

- It is a chronic disease.
- MS is unpredictable.
- Having MS is expensive.
- There are many emotional issues connected to MS.

You will probably want to share the fact that you have MS with your family members, and they may accept your information in different ways. Certainly it is best to share this information with the people closest to you. In telling family members you need to be in control and let them know that you are the same person they have always known and loved. You probably had MS before your diagnosis and functioned well. You may want to remind family members of this fact.

> *My mom and I have always been very close. I am married now, with two little ones, but my parents are only an hour away. My mom and I are still close and find time to do things together. I didn't know how Mom would take my diagnosis of MS. It took awhile for her to accept the fact that she and my father had done nothing to cause MS. Then Mom began to shower me with her help. She would appear wanting to clean my house or shop for me and constantly wanting to know what she could do for me. I finally decided that I could not live with too much help. I am fine, and I need to be able to live my life. I suggested to Mom that I really would appreciate her making a casserole for our freezer now and then. Mom loves to cook and is wonderful at it. She now comes over every other week or so with wonderful things for our freezer that the family so loves. I have told her over and over that "that is the kind of help we need."* FELICE

If you are a young person who must tell your parents that you have MS, they are very likely to feel that this is something they may have caused, and they may feel guilty. Their reaction may be to shower you with more help than you could ever want. Too much help can be very uncomfortable for you. On the other hand, if your parents are elderly, they may be so involved in their own activities that they ignore your information. That can be uncomfortable for you as well. Parents may not be able to deal with the reality of your diagnosis and may choose to ignore what you have told them, thinking that if they refuse to accept it it will go away. Let your parents know that they did not do anything that would have caused your diagnosis.

If you were very young when diagnosed, your parents, and not you, may have been told of the diagnosis. With pediatric MS being brought to light, more children are now being diagnosed than in years past. Parents sometimes wonder if they should delay telling their child about the diagnosis of MS. There are many reasons why this is not a good idea. First, open and honest communication promotes trust. Children will know they are sick, and they can often sense their parents' state of mind. This may lead them to speculate that something much, much scarier is going on. Also, in a best-care scenario, children should be included in their medical care decisions.

Disclosing Your Multiple Sclerosis Status to Your Children

MS is a chronic and unpredictable disease. It affects not just the person who has it but everyone around that person. Children are often worried about their parents and fear that a parent will become very disabled or will die. Some children may feel ashamed and embarrassed to go out in public with a parent who is visibly disabled and uses a wheelchair. Kids can be frustrated if you are unable to keep up with them or go to their school events or be involved in their activities. All of these reactions are normal. Fortunately, children do learn to adapt, and if adapting proves to be a problem, family counseling can help. There is no shame connected with needing help, and it is best that you deal with problems now rather than later.

Parents who have MS generally agree that their children adequately cope with the higher stress levels in their home. However, you should never underestimate the impact that living

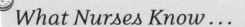

What Nurses Know...

MS affects the total family dynamic and cannot be tucked into the back of a closet. If it comes out before you have disclosed it, this may greatly change the level of trust in the family.

with a parent with a chronic illness can have on a child. Family counseling can be a valuable tool to help people cope with the unavoidable stress that comes with a diagnosis of MS.

Talking openly with children about MS can relieve their anxiety about their parent's health and their own security and what this means to them. If no explanation is given, children may use their vivid imaginations to come up with something much worse than what the reality is.

I was a great baseball player when I was a kid. I used to dream of being a professional player. I wasn't really good enough for that and ended up becoming a lawyer but always figured I would coach my son's baseball team. MS entered the picture for me, and I was unable to coach using my walker and my wheelchair, but I could make it to most of my son's games and discuss what had gone on. One day my boy will be able to coach his son's team. Meanwhile I am able to coach his homework and still be his dad. ROY

I guess I came from a "different" family. My mom had MS. She couldn't do all the things that other moms did, but she did different and very special other things. All my friends used to love to come to our house. When we were little, Mom told us stories, and as we grew older Mom helped us all with our homework and "girl talk." She had time that she devoted to us that other moms didn't. We are older now, but my friends still keep up with Mom. She is a very special person and a very special mom. SALLI-JO

What Nurses Know...

Having MS doesn't mean that you cannot be that special parent.

How Do You Tell Your Children?

When children have a better idea of what is going on they are less likely to feel like victims and more likely to feel "part of" of things. Honesty promotes trust and confidence, and that is important. The following are some tips for telling your child or children that you have been diagnosed with MS:

- Tailor the information to their age.
- Choose a time of day when they aren't tired or distracted.
- Don't feel you have to tell them everything about MS all at once. Tell them what they can handle based on their age, state the basics, and then answer any questions they have.
- Use real medical terms, and explain them to the best of your capacity.
- Express confidence in the doctors, and try to instill a positive outlook on your condition.
- It's OK to say "I don't know, but I'll try to find out" in reply to any question.
- Explain what changes your MS may make to your child's routine, if any.
- Leave the door open for them to come to you at any time with questions or concerns.

If there is a chapter of the National MS Society near you, get to know the members, and find out when they might be having family programs. It will be meaningful for your children to have friends who know what it is like to have MS as a part of the family.

Friends

Deciding which friends to tell is another decision you have to make. People react to illness in different ways. Some people are not able to accept illness and may drift away from you. However, others, some of whom you may not have been so close to before, may step up and be there for you as very special supporting friends. In deciding whom to tell you need to remember that very often people feel excluded and not trusted when they are not told about something or learn that something has been kept secret from them. Remember that they probably don't know any more about MS than you did when you were diagnosed. Tell your friends the diagnosis and prognosis. Let them know that MS is not contagious, that they cannot "catch" it from you. Let them think about it. Remind them that you're still you.

Also, you should consider that, aside from family members, other people can be called on to help, may even want to help.

Disclosing Your Diagnosis in the Workplace

You also will need to decide whether to tell people at your workplace that you have MS. This is a personal choice and completely up to you. If you have missed lots of work because of testing during your diagnosis, you may want to let your boss know what has happened, particularly if he or she is an understanding person. You may decide to be open about your diagnosis so that if sometime in the future you need some reasonable accommodations, such as working at home a few days a week, you will be more likely to get them. Meanwhile, you will show that you are the same person you were before you shared your diagnosis. Should you find that you do indeed need some changes to be able to do your job, you can request reasonable accommodations. You might find that if you could park close to where you work, you would not have to expend a great deal of energy to get into the office and thus be able to accomplish more at work. Asking for a handicapped place to park would be a reasonable accommodation. Your doctor will be willing to fill out a request for you to have a handicapped parking tag for your automobile. This might make a big difference when you go to a grocery store or shopping center by making it possible for you to park close to the front door so you have strength to shop once inside the store. If fatigue is a serious problem for you, you might request to work from home one or two days each week so that you could work on your own schedule on those days and not need to commute. Many people who have MS have found that their employer will make this kind of accommodation in order to keep a good employee.

> *I so love my job. I have been working at the same place for the past fifteen years. I love my boss and all of the people with whom I work, but the fatigue associated with my MS has increased, and I am good for absolutely nothing once I make it home from work. I thought about asking to go part time, but I need my full salary in order to live and I need to work full time in order to keep my insurance. My boss, when I finally worked up the courage to talk about my problem, suggested that I work from home two days each week. I am so grateful. On Tuesdays and Thursdays I have no commute and I am able to fit little rest periods into my day when I need them. Being able to do this has made a real difference in my week, my work, and my MS.* AGNES

If and when you choose to disclose your diagnosis to your boss and fellow employees, you may want to come prepared with a short fact sheet on MS. You can give them a brief piece of literature or offer to view some Web sites with them so that they can get an overview of exactly what MS is and what it isn't.

It is a good idea to prepare yourself with how you will cope with symptoms at work. If your MS causes you to forget things, use your personal tips and tricks for remembering things. It could be written instructions, Post-It notes, or color-coded reminders. If fatigue is an issue, you may want to consider a midday nap in a dark, quiet space or relaxation techniques you can do at your desk to rejuvenate yourself. You may close your eyes and just relax all of the muscles in your body for ten minutes or meditate on something peaceful for a few minutes.

MS, like all disabilities, is covered under the Americans with Disabilities Act, which gives civil rights protections to individuals with disabilities similar to those provided to individuals on the basis of race, color, sex, national origin, age, and religion. It guarantees equal opportunity for individuals with disabilities in public accommodations, employment, transportation, state and local government services, and telecommunications. If you have been officially diagnosed with MS, you have legal protections to fall back on should you believe discrimination has occurred.

I remember one person with MS who long ago decided not to share that fact at his workplace. Twenty years later, he was experiencing some progression in his disease and ended up telling the man in the cubicle next to him that he had MS. His cubicle neighbor informed him that he, too, had MS. All that time, they had been working side by side, never speaking of their shared illness.

Another young gal, newly diagnosed, went back to work and told her fellow workers about her diagnosis. They listened to her and then went about doing everything they could for her. They brought her drinks of water and wanted to bring her lunch. She came back to our support group not knowing what to do about all this. The group members told her to tell her friends how much it meant to her that they would want to do these things for her but that she was able to, and wanted to, take care of her own needs but that it meant so much to her to know that she could call on them if and when she needed their help.

When I was first diagnosed with MS, I decided that I would just keep it to myself and not tell anyone at work. Then one day I forgot and mentioned to my friend Bev that I had MS. She was great and didn't make a big thing of it. The National MS Society has a walk for MS every April, but I had no reason to be involved in that. Then Bev asked me to be a part of the walk. She had sent out a sign-up list for walkers to all of the people at work, and she had 105 people walking for me "Team Karen." I just couldn't believe that all of these people would walk for me! KAREN

I was recently diagnosed with MS, and I am only 23 years old. I want a life! I want to date. Do I have to tell everyone that I am no longer perfect? Don't date me! FRAN

MS is the most common neurological disease among young adults. Young adults are graduating from school, starting careers, and dating. They are sure that they are perfect, and they are not ready to tolerate something chronic like MS, which they fear will change everything. You do not need to wear a sign that says "I have MS, so don't come near me." You don't need to advertise the fact that you have MS. If you date someone long enough to have a relationship that may become serious, the fact that you have MS will probably have come out in a more casual way that does not require a big announcement. Certainly, if you are considering a permanent relationship or a marriage, the part MS could play needs to be considered. Your partner needs to understand MS and the fact that you hope to have a "normal" life but that it is not a predictable disease and is not symptom free. MS is definitely a part of who you are and will have a presence in your family life. "Normal" for you could be a little bit different than the "normal" anticipated before your diagnosis. The partner of a person with MS needs to understand that he or she will likely need to be able to provide support that they had not anticipated. Family life could be different, with role changes necessary. Being able to communicate verbally and nonverbally is all important. Include your partner in a visit to your MS provider or MS center. Involve him or her in a support group and in a serious talk with your doctor or MS nurse just so that you both have explored all of the possibilities of what could be ahead. You and your partner can work out how you will manage your family together and

What Nurses Know...

Years ago, women with MS were discouraged from having children. Doctors believed that pregnancy could make the disease worse and that afterward these women would not be able to care for young children. It's a different story nowadays. Studies have shown that pregnancy is actually protective for women with MS.

determine roles for each member, remembering the importance of open communication and trust.

Having MS does not mean that you cannot decide to have children. Women usually feel great during pregnancy. Health care professionals think that the role estrogen plays seems to protect women during pregnancy, and the role of estrogen in MS is currently being studied.

A women needs to cease her immunotherapy when planning a pregnancy and during the pregnancy and then restart it after the baby comes or after she finishes breast-feeding. Relapses are sometimes noted to be more frequent right after pregnancy. I like to think that a good reason for this might be having to be up with the baby at night. I often suggest to patients that the dad take over doing that and that the mom rests when the baby sleeps during the day. As a child grows up, the dad may have to do more things in the home. I mention "dad" because three quarters of individuals with MS are women, but the situation can certainly be reversed. In an MS family kids may learn to take on more jobs at an early age, when it is kind of fun to be permitted to do things like laundry and putting clothes away. They can learn to cook when their peers haven't had that opportunity, and it can be fun to "one up" them.

I remember one mom who had three children, all in after-school sports, and she just was not able to take them to practices. However, she was able to spend Mondays baking cookies, which she gave to the moms who drove the kids and didn't have time to bake. That absolved any guilty feelings she had for not driving, the driver families loved her, and her kids were proud of their mom.

Another decision that must be made is *how* to share MS with your children. As I stated earlier, I think it is important for kids to know that their parent has MS. They are very observant and will have a sixth sense that something is not right in the family. If you do not tell them yourself you run the risk that they will find out from someone other than you. A child may feel guilty and believe that he or she caused the MS. You must prepare the groundwork and keep up with good parent-child communication in the family. It is also probably important under most circumstances to let your children's teachers know about your diagnosis. They can be helpful in gauging how your children are responding to your illness.

The visible and invisible symptoms of MS can cause confusion and anger that lead to family disruption. People with MS and their family members may experience grief, anxiety, and/or resentment over their loss of control. A person who has MS feels guilty of possibly not being able to fulfill roles and responsibilities, and family members can feel guilty that they are not the

What Nurses Know...

MS always impacts the family. Each family has its own set of dynamics and its own rhythm, its own cultural, ethnic, and socioeconomic mores, and all of these are affected by a chronic illness.

one who has been diagnosed with a chronic illness. There can be many uncomfortable feelings. Inflammation can occur not only physically, in the central nervous system, but also metaphorically, in a person's reaction to the disease as well as in the form of disruptions in the family system. Individuals with MS and their families must respond to change and make choices that can cause stress when they realize that the seemingly limitless options of the past are no longer all feasible. Lots of things can interfere with family communication. Family members can become protective of their family member who has MS. They may be embarrassed. Most important of all, just because a group of people are members of a family does not mean that each family member copes with things in the same way. All of these things need to be considered by your health care team when you have MS. Your family needs to be involved in planning your treatment so that they can be a part of the goals you have established.

Sexuality

Sexuality is a complex and very important part of our lives. It goes far beyond the sex act itself. There is a part in each of us that is sexual. We interact with people of the same or opposite sex, communicating in a sexual way, and regardless of our abilities and disabilities we are all sexual beings. *Sexuality* can be defined as friendship, sharing and understanding, and as a way a person thinks and acts toward others. It affects your basic feelings of self-esteem and how you view yourself. *Intimacy* is that which is close or personal and the ability to share that with another. It is a feeling of belonging together and sharing affection or pleasure. Changes in sexuality may occur as a result of MS because of both physical and psychological difficulties. More than ninety percent of all men with MS and more than seventy percent of all women with MS report some change in their sexual life after the onset of the disease (Schapiro, 2003). These problems may be intermittent, and they may not be related to MS. A problem may not be a dysfunction but may be *perceived* as a dysfunction. A couple may have sexual problems because they no longer communicate with each other or they are angry with each other and that is not due to one partner having MS. They may not have been intimate before MS entered their relationship.

In Chapter 4 I discussed some of the changes that occur in the sexual lives of people with MS. Men often report impaired genital sensation, inability to achieve an erection, and delayed ejaculation. Women report impaired genital sensation, diminished organism, loss of sexual interest, diminished vaginal lubrication, and weak vaginal muscles. MS-related sexual dysfunction may be characterized as *primary, secondary,* or *tertiary.* Primary problems are directly related to neurologic damage in the central nervous system. These would include erectile and ejaculatory dysfunction, loss of lubrication, loss of sensation, decreased libido, and loss of orgasm. Sexual dysfunction characterized as secondary includes physical problems caused by MS that affect the human sexual response cycle. Secondary problems would include fatigue, spasticity, weakness, bowel and bladder problems, and cognitive problems. Last, MS-related sexual problems may be tertiary, comprising factors that affect an individual both psychologically and socially and interfere with the human sexual response. Tertiary problems might include depression, low self-esteem, role changes, poor communication, negative changes in self-image or body image, anger, guilt, feelings of isolation, or feelings of dependency.

Our sex life was great before MS, but now I am just too tired once it is finally time to go to bed. My fatigue, as well as the fact that I just don't feel as desirable as before, created a real problem between my husband and me. I finally actually talked with my neurologist about this and he really understood and suggested that we examine our schedules and make time for intimate time together at earlier times during the day or first thing in the morning. That worked for us. With just a few changes we feel like the couple we were before. ANNE

People with multiple sclerosis are prescribed medications to manage their MS symptoms or to control other medical problems that have nothing to do with their MS, and these medications can affect sexual function. Problems of decreased desire can be caused by psychoactive medications, such as antidepressants; or by some antihypertensives and cardiovascular medications; or even by very commonly used medications such as Dilantin, Pepcid, and Zantac. Psychoactive medications and antihypertensives can cause arousal disorders. Many of the same drugs that cause problems with desire also can cause orgasmic disorder that is the inablity to experience an organism.

In talking with people with MS when they come into the office I find that they very seldom mention that they are experiencing sexual problems. If I ask how they are doing, they may mention one of two symptoms or say that they are doing fine. If I then ask them about their sex life, I am likely to get a litany of problems followed by a statement that they feel they can't talk about those problems with the doctor. Sexual problems need to be shared with the doctor so that he or she can make changes in medications or arrange for professional counseling if necessary.

Sexuality and intimacy questionnaires are available to help determine where problems are so that they may be addressed. Good communication is critical to a positive sexual relationship but is something that many couples don't take the time to achieve. Couples need to be able to discuss honestly and openly what feels pleasurable. They need to learn now to express intimacy in their relationship. They need to understand sexual expression through cuddling, caressing, massage, and touch. They need to consider experimenting with a vibrator or other devices. Sexual expression can be adapted within the context of symptoms. Sexuality remains central in the lives of people with MS. Good communication between partners and good communication between the person with MS and his or her health care team is very important to a satisfying sexual life while living with MS. Sexual avoidance serves as a source of misunderstanding and emotional distress within a relationship. The person with MS may feel one or more of the following emotions:

- Denial
- Anxiety
- Fear and uncertainty
- Anger
- Guilt

Your partner may feel rejected and experience reduced self-esteem. Misunderstandings around this subject are common with MS and sometimes result in loss of desire or reduced emotional intimacy. So again, talk about it.

Relationships with other people will always be important. You had to relate to others before MS became a part of your life, and that will continue now that MS is a part of your life. MS is there, but don't let it be the center of your life. Whom to tell, how to tell them, and whether to tell them are all up to you. You still have to be the person you want to be. Changing the way you have done things in the past is not always bad and more often than not is a good thing.

Reference

Schapiro, RT. (2003). Managing the Symptoms of Multiple Sclerosis, Fourth Edition, New York, Demos Medical Publishing, 129-135.

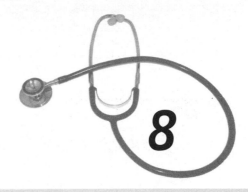

Taking Charge With a Chronic Disease

Living with multiple sclerosis (MS) is never going to be easy. I wouldn't have put MS on my list of things I want to have. It is difficult to have friends tell me how good I look when I am experiencing symptoms that make me feel not good at all but, in fact, make me feel terrible. It's hard to not know how I am going to be tomorrow. Then I stop to think about it. These things are on my mind because I know I have something chronic, but people who don't have chronic diseases really don't know what might happen to them tomorrow. I am going to learn all I need to know about MS, and then I am going to work to do everything I can to be the person I want to be.   PAULA

Webster's dictionary defines *hope* as a feeling "that what is wanted will happen; desire or accomplishment by expectation" and defines *hopeful* as "a feeling of showing hope." Hope is an anticipation of a future that is good. Hope is being positive and

What Nurses Know . . .

Having a diagnosis of MS may not be the end of your world. It can serve as a new beginning when you look at what you do differently and take the time to enjoy things you might not have considered before your diagnosis.

experiencing a sense of unlimited possibility and potential. Hope is something essential for a person with multiple sclerosis (MS) who is taking charge of his or her life with this chronic disease. Hopeful people accept the fact that they have MS and then learn all that they can about this disease. They do what they can to live the best life possible and put that knowledge to work in living life. This doesn't mean making MS the focal point of your life but rather tucking away what you learn and using that information when needed.

People with MS learn that not everything about this disease is bad. I remember speaking to a woman who had had MS for many years and came into the office in a wheelchair. This was before any immunotherapies for MS were available. I was a new MS nurse and said something to her about how difficult life must be for her. She looked up and told me that not everything about MS was bad. She said that, for instance, she and her husband had planned when they got married to set aside money they might spend for vacations and save to take a trip around the world once their children were grown. They had three children when she was diagnosed with MS. She and her husband felt the uncertainty of MS and decided that they would forget waiting for a trip together around the world and instead would have some kind of a vacation each year with the family. This lady sitting there in her wheelchair told me that she felt thankful to MS. She said that

What Nurses Know...

"Attitude is a little thing that makes a big difference."
—Winston Churchill

her family has the most wonderful memories of their vacations together. Family life took on a new meaning, a bond that she and her children and husband would not have experienced were it not for MS. You may not experience something as dramatic as my friend here did, but as you live your life you probably will see things that you did differently because of MS and come to understand that some of those differences had a positive influence on your life. Your challenge is to be able to note these things and be grateful for them.

We humans can be so definite about the things in our lives that we shall and shall not accept. How many times do we say that we will "never" do this or that? As a parent, I have said something like that so many times and ended up eating my words. Myrna was a gal in a support group which I ran who said over and over that there was one thing that she would never use, and that was a wheelchair. To her, a wheelchair was the picture of utter defeat. One holiday season we were talking about ways to get ready for the holidays, and Myrna went on about how exhausted trying to shop made her. She could head to a store and buy one thing and be so exhausted that she had to head for the car and home. I suggested that she just try using one of the wheelchairs available at the shopping center. She let me know that there was no way she would do that! At our next meeting Myrna spoke up and said that she had to "eat crow." She told us that, after much thought, she had decided to try the wheelchair at the shopping center. Her husband wheeled, and she shopped and held the packages. She said that they got so much done and that she was able to enjoy going out to dinner on the way home. Myrna and her husband decided to get a lightweight wheelchair just to use for special travel times. They took the family to Disney World with Myrna in her chair, and Myrna said she gained new respect from her three teenagers when her wheelchair permitted them all to go to the front of the lines.

Things like holiday shopping, and shopping in general, can be frustrating when you have MS fatigue. Using the Internet and catalogs can make a real difference in getting it done and limiting time spent at the mall. You also can look into other perks that are available to people with chronic disease, such as half-price theater tickets. And don't forget the handicapped parking tag that you can have for your car to use when you need it (see Chapter 7).

We live in Washington, DC, and my husband and I loved being able to see special presentations at the Kennedy Center. A few years ago my husband was diagnosed with MS and cut back on his work time. I continued to work part time as well, but we just didn't have funds for things like trips to the Kennedy Center. Someone in our support group told us that we could qualify for half-price tickets. We can get out again and do something that we both love. What a difference that makes in both of our lives!   PHYLLIS

Hugo Schwartz had had MS for twenty-five years when I first met him several years ago. He was one of the hardest working men I have known. His MS made ambulation very difficult for him, but he never missed a day of work. He came into our office for his medical visits using two canes and out of energy. He used those canes to get from his car to his office, and from the office to the bathroom, and he ate his lunch at his desk. Hugo had moved to this country years before from Germany, and he and his wife would make a trip back home to visit family in Germany every couple of years. Proud as he was, Hugo finally agreed to a wheelchair at the airport for these trips. My colleagues and I kept telling him how much easier his life would be if he would just purchase and use a scooter. He would have more energy for work, and getting around at home–and certainly visits with his family in Germany–would be so much easier if he were to use a scooter. We had given up, when one day Hugo appeared for his appointment driving a bright red scooter. He had a smile wide on his face and looked up and said that things were much easier now. He thanked us for the suggestion. Assistive devices, should you need them, can enable you to live a much better life.

Assistive devices that may make a difference in your life with MS might include one or more of the following:

- An ankle-foot orthosis, which is designed to help you walk by decreasing spasticity. It tilts the foot to a specified angle to keep it from turning in or out, thus decreasing fatigue and increasing stability.
- A cane, leg braces, or a crutch, which can help you improve mobility.
- A walker, which can help with balance. One with wheels and a seat can help with fatigue.
- A wheelchair, standard or electric, which can offer independence.
- A scooter, which can bring independence and can be taken apart to travel in a car.

- Reacher devices, if you have trouble bending or reaching things.
- Grab bars and handrails installed in your bathtub and shower areas, which provide support to help you maintain balance.

I have MS. I have been doing really well, but I reached a point when my physical therapist suggested that I begin using a cane. I didn't have a problem learning to use the cane, but I just hated to have that ugly thing with me. I need to mention that I am fortunate enough to have a wonderful help dog who helps me with everything. My friend borrowed my cane for a couple of days and brought it back having painted pictures of my dog all over the cane. Now I have two conversation pieces: my wonderful dog and my cane.   IRMA

Something that can be very difficult when you have MS is accepting assistance from others. This is particularly difficult when you have always been the one to do the assisting. It is always easier to do something for someone else than it is to let someone do for you. A friend of mind, Paula, learned this lesson quite by accident. Paula and her husband loved to entertain friends and always had Thanksgiving with all of the trimmings at their home. They did everything themselves, and their guests were truly guests. Paula has MS. One Thanksgiving she was hit with a bad exacerbation. She could barely get herself out of bed, and there was Thanksgiving dinner for twelve to be prepared. Guests were scheduled to come at 2:00 p.m. The guests

What Nurses Know . . .

It isn't easy either to ask for help or to realize that you have many friends who are anxious to be helpers.

arrived, and Paula took on a new role, that of sitting back and giving directions to everyone else. Dinner was a little later than planned, but it was wonderful. All of the guests had the time of their lives cooking and fixing the food. They begged Paula to let them do this every year, and it has become a new tradition. Paula told me that this experience has changed her life. She realizes that friends really do want to help and that together they can have many more good times. Being able to accept assistance is a good thing all around.

Healthy Living With MS

One of the things that it is so easy to do when you have a chronic condition like MS is to blame MS for everything that happens to you. You have to be careful! As I have stated earlier, a diagnosis of MS does not provide immunity from all other illnesses, and MS is not the cause of all your problems. People with MS need regular physical examinations. You need the amount of sleep that your body requires. You need to maintain a healthy diet and weight control. You need to keep vaccinations up to date, and you need regular exercise. You need to do all of the things that bring about good, healthy living.

In your thirties you should have a physical exam every three to four years to check for hypertension, the beginning of heart disease, and cancer. In your forties you need to schedule a

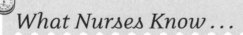

What Nurses Know . . .

Healthy living is a must when you have MS—even more so than for people who do not have a chronic illness. Take care of your body and your mind with satisfying personal relationships, a strong support network, a fulfilling job, fun hobbies, and attention to your inner self.

physical exam every two years and watch that cholesterol level. Men need a digital rectal exam, and women need annual breast and pelvic exams with a pap smear and a mammogram every one to two years. You may require an electrocardiogram and stress test. In your fifties you need yearly physical exams to check for hypertension, arteriosclerosis, cancer, diabetes, arthritis, and bronchial conditions, as well as a colonoscopy to be repeated every ten years if the first one is negative and you have no family history of colon cancer. In your sixties and later you need the same type of physical exam as you did in your fifties, with hearing and vision tests added yearly. People with MS who have used steroids need to have regular bone density tests. Immunizations should be given when your MS is stable and you are not in the midst of an exacerbation—generally four to six weeks after the last dose of steroid. Vaccines considered safe for people with MS include the influenza vaccination as well as those for Hepatitis B, varicella (chicken pox), tetanus, shingles, and pneumococcus. The tuberculosis test also is considered safe for people with MS. An MMR (measles-mumps-rubella) vaccination is probably safe, but serologic testing should be done first to check for need. For other vaccinations, such as polio, typhoid, and yellow fever, published evidence is inconclusive, but if you will be going to a country where they are required you will need to have them.

Again, healthy living is an absolute requirement for anyone with MS. Make time for exercise. Proper exercise increases fitness and reduces fatigue. A physical therapist or personal trainer who knows MS can develop exercise programs specifically for you; they will show you the right type of exercise, how long you should exercise, how often you should exercise, and how hard you should exercise. I find that for young people today exercise is such an important part of their lives that they are relieved to know that they need to keep it up. Older people who haven't been used to exercise find it a little more difficult to make it a part of their lives but must be encouraged to do so.

I never have liked to exercise, and as I became older I found
excuse after excuse not to do it. Then came MS. I decided

that I would walk every day, until I began to have problems with balance. My therapist suggested that I try exercising in a swimming pool and arranged for me to be part of an exercise group at a pool not far from home. I can do so much in the water with no fatigue and I feel so good about myself afterward.   SHERRY

You need to learn to manage stress. Realistically, stress can't be avoided, but you can learn ways to manage the unavoidable, and you can use relaxation techniques such as meditation, guided imagery, spirituality, prayer, and exercise. Yoga and tai chi can help mix exercise and spirituality. You can make your home user friendly by arranging things so that items you use often are easily reached and you will be able to sit while you do tasks. Your doctor can arrange for an occupational therapy evaluation so you can learn how to make your home user friendly for someone with disability. Something as simple as a stool in the kitchen to be used when preparing meals can help fatigue. You can teach your family to share tasks of daily living, and you can work to improve family communication and sharing of tasks. You need to plan for the worst situations and hope for the best. If you are building a home or planning renovations to your existing home, arrange for wider door openings and wider showers. You may never need them, but they will be there should you eventually need them.

What Nurses Know . . .

The right exercise can make a real difference in how you function and how you feel about yourself. Try different things to find out what you really like. It is definitely worth the time and effort on your part.

What Nurses Know...

According to a study published in the journal Neurology, just six months of yoga significantly reduced fatigue in people with MS (Oken BS, Kishiyama MA, Zajdel D. et al, 2010).

Another thing you need to do is to look at your diet and nutrition. There is no conclusive evidence that any particular nutritional therapy affects the course of MS. Almost every newly diagnosed person with MS asks if there is an MS diet. It would be wonderful to be able to control the disease with a diet, but no diets have yet been proven to control MS at this point in time. I discussed nutrition and diet in Chapter 6, but it is such an important topic that I need to mention again that sensible eating habits have a dramatic beneficial impact on many other aspects of health and are important for everyone, especially individuals with a chronic illness.

I also need to repeat once again that obtaining a healthy body weight, along with good nutrition, is crucial, because steroid use and other medications used in MS, plus physical disabilities, can foster weight gain, as can a sedentary lifestyle. You need proper portion size, a wide variety of foods that are high in complex carbohydrates, and a wide variety of vegetables and fruits each day. You need to cut back on saturated fat and reduce your intake of simple sugar such as cookies, cakes, candy, and desserts. Eat fish regularly. Drink more water and less soda, as well as fewer sweetened beverages and beverages high in caffeine. Limit salt and learn to read nutrition labels. Add vitamin supplements when suggested by your health care provider. Your health care team can suggest someone to help you with nutrition if you need assistance. Good general health means limiting alcohol intake and not smoking. If you are a smoker, get help to stop and *stop.* Smoking does not help general health, and it does not help MS!

Support Groups

Join a support group if there is one in your area. Find a good one that is positive and not a gripe session. Look for one that is led by someone who knows MS. If your local MS center does not have such a group, see if the National MS Society sponsors a group in your area. Not everyone is ready to accept their MS or is ready for a support group, but if you can overcome your initial resistance and keep attending it, you may note a real change in your attitude toward your disease. A support group provides information about MS and keeps you up to date on current MS research. It provides you with a particular time to focus on the topic, so you don't need to constantly think about MS as you live the other days of your life. It is comforting to be with other people who understand how you feel and who have been where you were, or are where you are. A support group will give you an opportunity to share how you handle problems, get feedback from others, and form lasting friendships. Family members can go with you and learn to understand MS.

The last thing I wanted to have suggested to me when I was diagnosed with this disease was that I join a support

What Nurses Know...

Support groups can make life with MS so much better by increasing your knowledge about the disease and giving you the opportunity to see how other people handle the same issues you confront.

group. Support groups aren't for me! I didn't want to be with people in wheelchairs and hear them gripe. My center had a group devoted to newly diagnosed patients. With lots of urging from the staff there I decided to go to just one meeting. I have to say that it was a real surprise. My MS doctor and MS nurse led the meeting. It was like having a free hour and a half with my doctor. There was no griping. I got lots of information even though I had decided I didn't need it. Everyone there was normal, just like me. I decided to come back to the ten monthly sessions that the group had, and I brought my girlfriend. Now I know that I am on the right track, and I don't make my MS the focus of my life. I still don't like the word "support group," but the people in this group became special to me.   SAM

Online Support

You will find support at good Internet sites such as those of the National MS Society, the Multiple Sclerosis Association of America, the Eastern Paralyzed Veterans Association, the Multiple Sclerosis Society of Canada, and the Consortium of Multiple Sclerosis Centers, which are listed in the Resources section at the back of this book along with other helpful sites. You will want to look into the North American Research Committee on Multiple Sclerosis (NARCOMS), which was developed in 1993 by the Consortium of Multiple Sclerosis Centers as a confidential way to provide detailed information about yourself and the course and treatment of your disease for research purposes. This registry is free, and participation provides you with a free subscription to the *Multiple Sclerosis Quarterly Report*; notification of clinical trials for which you might be eligible, with no obligation; and an invitation to complete surveys for other MS research projects. In the Resources section of this book you will find contact information for the pharmaceutical support organizations that provide the therapies used for the various MS research projects

There are many online methods of support for all of you who search the Internet. It is important that you pick positive Web sites. There are gripe sessions out there, and they are not a good place to be. The National MS Society Web site (www. nationalmssociety.org) is probably the most visited site for information about MS and is a great place to start. All of the immunotherapies you take have good, helpful Web sites, and you should feel free to use them all, not just the one for the drug you are taking. I used to try to keep a list of good Web sites a the MS center where I work, but it got so that there were so many that I could not be all inclusive. Lots of people with MS have found real support through the Internet, and many have formed lasting friendships with some of the people with whom they correspond. With the rise of the Internet, millions are turning to online peer support groups for health support. If you feel you need to talk with others with MS, about the everyday challenges they have to deal with, medical treatments, parenting, relationships—really, anything—you may enjoy an online group. There is a give-and-take nature about groups that becomes helpful for all involved. If you would like some advice and good ideas on managing your illness, why not give online peer support a try? Another thing that online support has going for it is it is truly accessible for all. You don't need to leave your house. Also, you can get real-time support in your time of need. The free exchange, the mutual giving

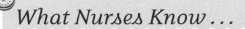

What Nurses Know ...

You must live for today but hope for tomorrow and know what has come before.

and receiving of support, is the essence of any peer support group. The following are some places to start to collect information and contacts:

- www.facebook.com
- www.msfriends.org
- ms.about.com
- www.patientslikeme.com
- www.msworld.org
- www.dailystrength.org

Those are just a starting point. Get out there and write a blog. Share your experience!

I had a very special MS nurse friend, Linda Morgante, from the Maimonides MS Center in New York, who conducted research on the importance of hope for people with MS. She shared her work with the rest of us as members of the International Organization of MS Nurses. We lost Linda to colon cancer a few years ago. At a memorial service in her honor little stones engraved in gold with the word *HOPE* were passed out. I put my "hope rock" on my dresser, where I see it each morning as I begin my day. It became such an important part of my life that I brought hope rocks for all of our MS patients in a program at our center so that they too would have reminders for their day. I am proud to

What Nurses Know...

I have learned that only special people have MS. What I haven't been able to determine is whether they were special before they had MS or if having MS made them special. I know that you are a very special person!

say that the Maimonides MS Center has changed its name to the Linda Morgante MS Center. Our friend Linda and her work on hope live on.

I began this chapter with a discussion of the importance of living with hope. Make hope a core part in your life. Hope for a cure for MS. Hope to be able to make the most of your life and the part that your MS plays in that life. Hope for the strength you need as you cope with life. Go for the very best quality of life. Become an active participant in the fight to cure MS.

Reference

Oken BS, Kishiyama MA, Zajdel D. et al. Randomized controlled trial of yoga and exercise in multiple sclerosis. *Neurology*, Arch Intern Med. 2010;170(4):321-331.

Glossary

Ankle-foot orthosis—A brace or splint used to support the foot by stabilizing it and tilting it to a specific angle to prevent spasticity

Anxiety—A feeling of worry, uneasiness.

Autoimmune disease—Disease such as rheumatoid arthritis or **multiple sclerosis** (MS) that involves the immune system of the body turning against a componet of the body itself.

Axons—The processes or extensions of nerve cells that conduct nervous impulses away from the cell body.

Bladder—Muscular sac that stores urine prior to urination.

Bowel—Lowest portion of the large intestine, involved in elimination.

Brain stem—The part of the **central nervous system** (CNS) that conrols breathing and the heart and connects the cerebrum to the spinal cord.

Bulk former—Substance that adds bulk to the stool.

Central nervous system—Consists of the brain and spinal cord. It is where many bodily functions, such as muscle control, eyesight, breathing, memory, and so forth, are generated, processed, and signaled to different parts of the body.

Cerebellum—The part of the brain responsible for coordinating motor movement.

Cerebrospinal fluid (CSF)—A clear fluid that surrounds and cushions the brain and spinal cord.

Cognition—Comprehension and use of speech; visual perceptions and construction; calculation ability; attention; information processing; memory; and executive functions such as planning, problem solving, and self-monitoring.

Colon—Lower part of the large intestine.

Constipation—Inability or difficulty in relieving oneself of stool.

Coping—Adjusting or adapting successfully to a challenge.

Demyelination—Abnormal process of myelin destruction that results in disruption of the normal pattern of nerve conduction.

Depression—Altered mood characterized by feelings of gloom.

Dendrite—The branched part of a nerve cell that carries impulses toward the cell body.

Dexamethasone—A high-potency cortisone used to decrease swelling or inflammation in the nervous system.

Ejaculation—Ejection of semen from the penis.

Evoked potentials—Stimulation of an organ (e.g., eye, ear, skin) to elicit an electrical discharge in the brain.

Exacerbation—Sudden worsening of symptoms. Also called a *relapse* or a *flare.*

Fatigue—A feeling of tiredness that in MS is often associated with a debilitating **lassitude.**

Gait–Walking pattern, often disrupted in MS.

Genetic–Pertaining to heredity.

Hereditary disease–One that is transmitted from one generation to another.

Immunosuppressant drug–Medication used to decrease the level of function of the immune system.

Immune system–Consists of a number of different organs in the human body (e.g., lymph nodes, bone marrow, thymus) that produce certain types of white blood cells and antibodies that have the ability to destroy or neutralize various germs, substances, poisons and other harmful substances.

Incontinence–Inability to control the bladder or bowels.

Incoordination–Inability to produce a harmonious, rhythmic muscular action that is not the result of weakness.

Interferon–A group of immune system proteins, produced and released by cells infected by a virus, that inhibit vital multiplication and modify the body's immune responses.

Intramuscular injection–Given with a 1- to 1½-inch needle into the muscle.

Lassitude–Specific type of fatigue occurring in MS characterized by a feeling of overwhelming tiredness.

Laxative–A food or chemical substance that acts to treat constipation.

Lesion–A physical abnormality in the nervous system. Also called a **plaque**.

Lumbar puncture–A **spinal tap**, involving the insertions of a needle into the spinal canal in order to obtain CSF.

Lyme disease–A recurrent inflammatory disorder characterized by distinctive skin rash, arthritis, and involvement of the heart and nervous system; caused by a spirochete and tickborn.

Magnetic resonance imaging– Diagnostic procedure that produces visual images of different body parts without the use of x rays. An important diagnostic tool in MS that makes it possible to visualize and count **lesions** in the white matter of the brain and spinal cord.

Monotherapy–Giving a treatment alone and not in combination with another treatment.

Myelin–A substance consisting of fat and protein, which acts as an insulator around most of the nerve fibers in the human body.

Naltrexone–An oral medication approved y the U.S. Food and Drug administration(FEA) for the treatment of opiate and alcohol addiction and proposed as effective in prevening MS attacks, slowing the progression of MS and treating MS symptoms.

Nerve–A bundle of nerve fibers (**axons**). Nerve fibers can lead toward the brain, serving in the perception of the sensory stimuli of skin, joins, muscles, and inner organs, or away from the brain, mediating contraction of muscles or organs.

Neurologist–A physician who specializes in the diagnosis and treatment of diseases of the nervous system.

Neuron–An individual nerve cell.

Numbness–Loss of sensation in an area of the body.

Nutrition–The body's use of food.

Oligoclonal bands–A diagnostic sign indicating abnormal levels of certain antibodies in the CSF seen in approximately ninety percent of people with MS, but not specific to MS.

Optic neuritis–Inflammation of the nerve that connects the eye with the brain, which manifests itself mainly as blurring or loss of vision and occasional pain.

Orgasm–The height of excitement a the time of sexual intercourse.

Orgasmic disorder—inability to have an orgasm during sexual intercourse.

Plaque–Area of inflamed or demyelinated CNS tissue. Also called a **lesion**.

Remission–A lessening in the severity of symptoms or their temporary disappearance during the course of an illness.

Sensory–Pertaining to the ability to feel, sense, taste, smell, see, and hear.

Sexuality–Related to the total sexual life of a person–whether including the sexual organs themselves or not.

Spasticity–Loss of normal elasticity of leg and/or arm muscles resulting from a disease process in the CNS. It is often manifested by extreme stiffness of the muscles, which results in difficulties with active and passive movements of the extremities.

Spinal cord–The part of the CNS that connects the brain and its related structures to the peripheral nervous system.

Spinal tap–See **Lumbar puncture**.

Steroids–Chemicals that either mimic or are from various endocrine organs of the body (usually the adrenal glands) that are potent anti-inflammatory and immune-suppressing agents often used in the management of MS.

Subcutaneous injection–An injection given by a 0.5-inch or ⅝-inch needle no deeper than 0.5 inch under the skin.

Symptom–The subjective description of a problem as perceived by the individual.

Titrate–To start with a small dose and gradually increase the dose to the amount needed.

Trigeminal neuralgia–Severe pain in the face due to irritation of a nerve from the brain stem.

Urethra–The canal for discharge of urine from the bladder.

Urinary tract–The pathway involved in urination; includes the kidney, ureter, bladder, and urethra.

Urine culture–The growing of bacteria from a specimen of urine to determine the presence and cause of infection.

Virus–Small organism with distinctive feature consisting of either DNA or RNA that is unaffected by most antibiotics and sometimes can be shown to be involved in some diseases.

Vitamin–A substance essential for growth, development, and normal body processes

Voiding–Elimination of urine or stool.

Weakness–A decrease in physical strength.

Resources

Books From Demos Health

Fishman, L. M., & Small, E. L. (2007). *Yoga and multiple sclerosis: a journey to health and healing.*

Gingold, J. (2006). *Facing the cognitive challenges of multiple sclerosis.*

Gingold, J. (2006). *Mental sharpening stones: manage the cognitive challenges of multiple sclerosis.*

Halper, J. (2009). *Living with progressive multiple sclerosis: overcoming the challenges* (2nd ed.).

Holland, N. (2007). *Multiple sclerosis: a guide for the newly diagnosed* (3rd ed.).

LaRocca, N., & Kalb, R. (2006). *Multiple sclerosis: understanding the cognitive challenges.*

Lowenstein, N. (2009). *Fighting fatigue in multiple sclerosis: practical ways to create new habits and increase your energy.*

Joffe, R., & Friedlander, J. (2008). *Women, work, and autoimmune disease: keep working, girlfriend!*

Kalb, R. (2008). *Multiple sclerosis: the questions you have—the answers you need* (4th ed.).

Kalb, R. (2006). *Multiple sclerosis: a guide for families* (3rd ed.).

Murray T. J. (2005). *Multiple sclerosis the history of a disease.*

Murray, T. J., & Bowling A. (2006). *Multiple sclerosis: the guide to treatment and management* (6th ed.).

Perkins, L. E., & Perkins, S. D. (2008). *Multiple sclerosis: your legal rights* (3rd ed.).

Peterman Schwarz, S. (2006). *Multiple sclerosis:300 tips for making life easier* (2nd ed.).

Robitaille, S. (2010). *The illustrated guide to assistive technology & devices: tools and gadgets for living independently.*

Schapiro, R. T. (2007). *Managing the symptoms of multiple sclerosis* (5th ed.).

Stachowiak, J. (2010). *The multiple sclerosis manifesto: action to take, principles to live by.*

Other Books

Blackstone, M. (2007). *Multiple sclerosis: an essential guide for the newly diagnosed.* Cambridge, MA: Da Capo Press.

Kalb, R., Holland, N., & Giesser, B. (2007). *Multiple sclerosis for dummies.* New York: For Dummies.

Lechtenberg, R. (1995). *Multiple sclerosis fact book* (2nd ed.). Philadelphia, PA: F. A. Davis.

Magazines

New Mobility. www.newmobility.com

MSFocus. www.msfocus.org/magazines-newsletters.aspx

Momentum. This great magazine is put out by the National Multiple Sclerosis Society. You can contact them directly for it: www.nationalmssociety.org

Organizations and General Interest

Can Do Multiple Sclerosis. www.mscando.org

Consortium of Multiple Sclerosis Centers. www.mscare.org

Eastern Paralyzed Veterans Association. www.epva.org

International Organization of MS Nurses. www.iomsn.org

MS Friends. www.msfriends.org

Multiple Sclerosis International Federation. www.msif.org
Multiple Sclerosis Foundation. www.msf.org
Multiple Sclerosis Association of America. www.msaa.com
Multiple Sclerosis Society of Canada. www.mssociety.ca
MS World. www.msworld.org
National Multiple Sclerosis Society. www.nationalmssociety.org
Paralyzed Veterans of America. www.pva.org
General Medical Information. www.webmd.com, www.about.com
Medicare Information. www.medicare.com

Pharmaceutical Company Web Sites

Bayer (manufacturer of betaseron). www.bayer.com
Biogen Idec (manufacturer of Avonex and Tysabri). www.biogen.
    com
EMD Serono (manufacturer of Rebif). www.serono.com/ms
Novartis (manufacturer of Gilenya and Extavia). www.novartis.
    com
Teva Neuroscience (manufacturer of Copaxone). www.tevaneuro-
    science.com

Index